THE POWER OF
REIKI

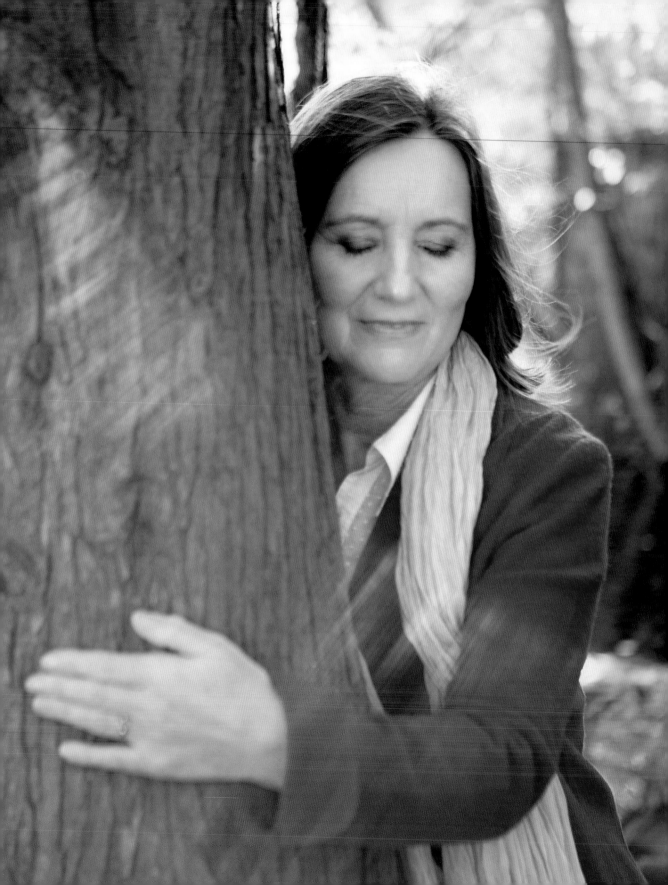

THE POWER OF
REIKI

An Ancient Hands-On Healing Technique

REIKI MASTER-TEACHER

TANMAYA HONERVOGT

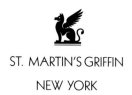

ST. MARTIN'S GRIFFIN

NEW YORK

www.stmartins.com

Library of Congress Cataloging-in-Publication Data Available Upon Request

ISBN 978-1-250-04948-3

St. Martin's Griffin books may be purchased for educational, business,
or promotional use. For information on bulk purchases, please contact
Macmillan Corpartate and Premium Sales Department at 1-800-221-7945,
extension 5442, or write specialmarkets@macmillan.com

Second U.S. Edition: April 2014

Originally published in Great Britain in 1998 by Gaia Books LTD

10 9 8 7 6 5 4 3 2 1

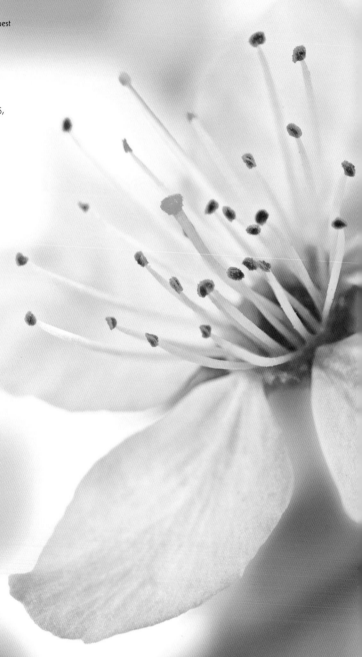

This book is dedicated to all seekers and healers for a fulfilled life, in harmony with themselves and all other beings on this planet.

"The function of the healer is to reconnect, but when I say the function of the healer is to reconnect, I don't mean that the healer has to do something. The healer is just a function. The doer is life itself, the whole."

Osho, *Beloved of my Heart*

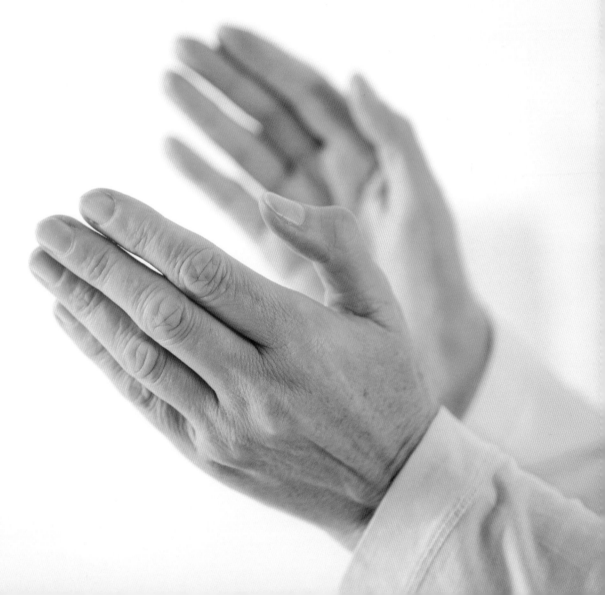

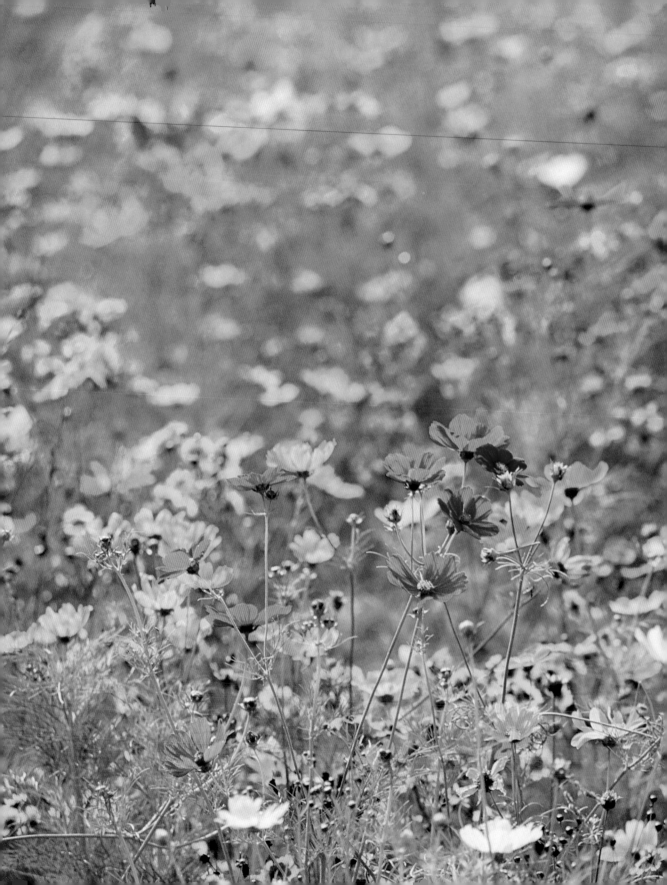

CONTENTS

ABOUT THIS BOOK

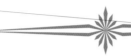

Reiki is a simple technique for transferring healing energy from a giver to a receiver. The word "Reiki" (pronounced "ray-key") means Universal Life Energy, and the ability to bring about healing during Reiki is gained through receiving attunements during a special initiation ceremony. The energy attunement opens a channel in the giver for more energy to flow through, to wherever it is most needed in the receiver. This can occur on a physical, mental, emotional, or spiritual level.

The attunements are given during First, Second, and Third Degree seminars, by a certified Master-Teacher. The unique Reiki Symbols with their mantras, which enable the Reiki power to work on a vibrational level, are handed on from Reiki Master to the student, in confidence, during the Second and Third Degree teachings. They are secret and are therefore not published in this book. However, the theory behind the use of the Symbols is fully explained.

This book is an introduction to the world of Reiki and is a resource and background book for Reiki Degree courses and seminars. It outlines the theory and history of Reiki and shows the hand positions that are taught, explaining how they are used for self-healing, for healing others, and for healing animals, plants, and the wider community. The book is also intended to be used as a visual inspiration for those who want to make Reiki an important part of their lives and for those who are already learning about it.

CAUTION

The exercises, hand positions, and meditations described in this book are intended for the healing and harmonization of living things. The author nevertheless wishes to point out that, in the case of illness, a doctor or healing practitioner should always be consulted. The Reiki positions described may naturally be applied as an additional form of treatment. Neither the author nor the publisher accept any responsibility for the application of the Reiki methods described in this book.

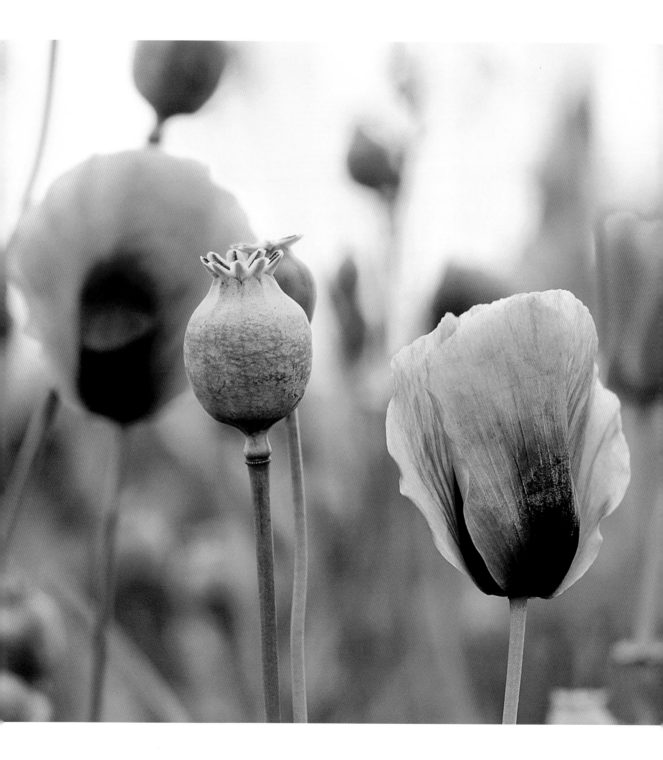

9

INTRODUCTION

"Until we know the state of your inner harmony, we can at the most release you from your illness – because your inner harmony is the source of your health. But when we release you from one illness, you will immediately catch another, because nothing has been done with regard to your inner harmony. The fact of the matter is that it is your inner harmony which must be supported."
Paracelsus, *Hidden Mysteries of Eastern Temples*

As Paracelsus says, the source of health is inner harmony. This book is intended to assist you on your path to becoming whole and to give you a practical guide to inviting healing and harmony into your life.

Reiki is an ancient healing method which is once again becoming known and popular in our modern age. It is a simple healing technique that is easy to learn and which can provide a real enrichment of your everyday life.

Reiki can be learned by anyone who opens him- or herself to it. Children can also be "initiated" in Reiki. Reiki offers you a wide-ranging insight into the various areas of the human experience – physical, mental, emotional, and spiritual. Reiki not only promotes your physical well-being but also has a positive effect on your emotional and spiritual equilibrium. This is why, after a treatment with Reiki, many people feel refreshed, relaxed, clearer, and more content in themselves.

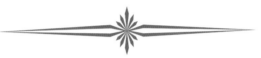

Reiki is suitable for healthy and sick people of all ages. You can use it to replenish your vital energy, to strengthen the immune system, and to ward off disease. At the same time, Reiki helps in the healing of ailments and illnesses such as headaches, body tensions, exhaustion, depression and fears, as well as acute and chronic disorders of all kinds. According to the writings of Dr Hayashi (see pp. 35–36), Reiki simultaneously treats the spiritual and mental causes of an illness, not merely the physical symptoms. The role of the symptom is to show us that something is not functioning properly in the body. You will learn through your practice of Reiki to regard the human being as a totality of body, soul, and mind and to treat all these levels as necessary.

I hope that this book will encourage you to explore your own life and that the practical exercises in it will vitalize, relax, and enrich

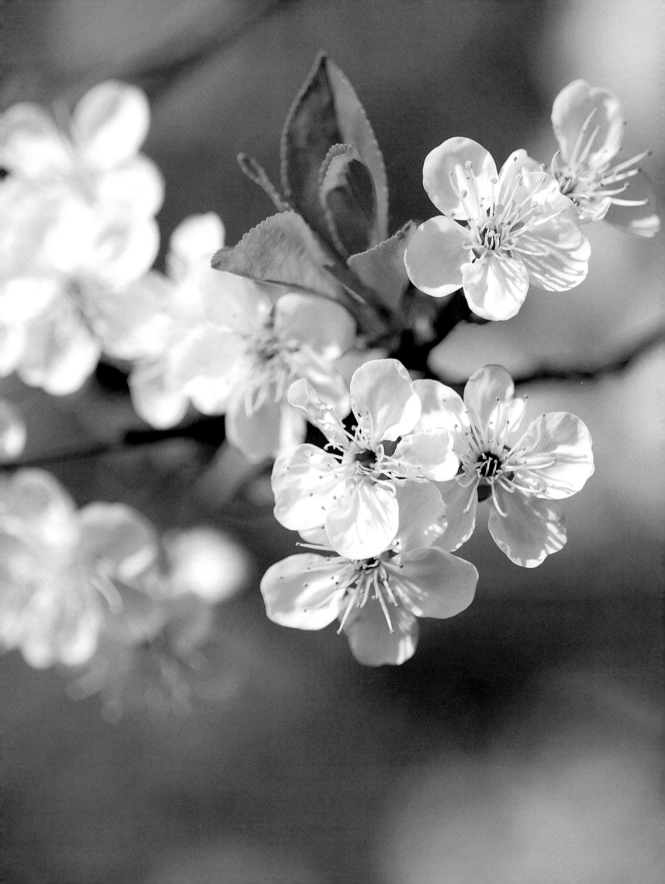

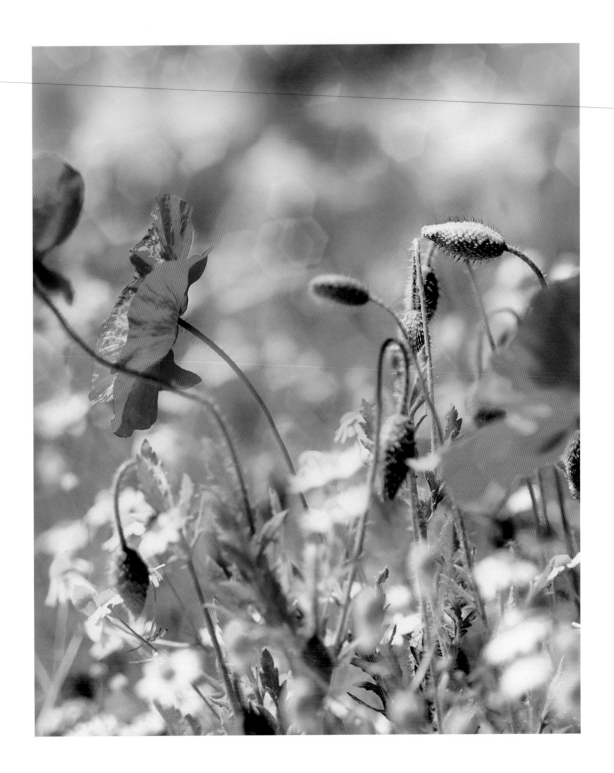

12

you. Reiki means self-healing and it assists you on your voyage of inward discovery. If you use Reiki every day, it will contribute appreciably to the renewal of your vital energy, to your healing, and to your physical and mental well-being. Have a lot of fun reading and experimenting and perhaps you will decide to become a "channel" for Universal Life Energy, known as Reiki.

I very much enjoyed writing this book and I realize now how much deeper it took me into Reiki. I discovered more and more about this fascinating healing method and all the different possibilities for using its energies.

Teaching Reiki has always been very rewarding and personally nourishing, so I would like to thank all my students for their support and for sharing their own experiences with me, and through this book with you also.

I hope that you enjoy reading this book and that you receive inspiration from it – whatever that may be and whatever you need in your life.

Tanmaya Honervogt

ABOUT THE AUTHOR

Tanmaya Honervogt holds regular training courses in the Reiki healing method and gives lectures and seminars both in Great Britain and overseas. She is the founder of the School of Usui Reiki (1995) in Devon, England.

Tanmaya regularly shares the latest developments of her healing work, seminars, healing meditations and much more. Visit her website, email her or subscribe to her newsletter or simply find Tanmaya on the Internet in order to find out more.

www.tanmaya-reiki.com

1. MY PATH
WITH REIKI

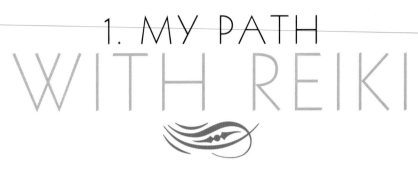

Reiki is a gift of the universe. As you grow with Reiki you will contribute healing and harmony to yourself and to your world. In the summer of 1983 I was on holiday in California, still ignorant of the wonderful healing art known as Reiki.

I was about thirty years old, and in the course of the previous eight years had taken part in several meditation courses and self-experience groups – an inward journey that had brought me a little nearer to myself. In Germany I had worked as a teacher, but had failed to find personal fulfillment.

I felt drawn to learning to do some form of hands-on healing. I had become aware that there was something in my hands that needed to express itself, but I did not know what it was. I knew I had to realize a hidden potential – a latent possibility – and was searching for a way to let it come out. At that point I had massage or shiatsu in mind because I was familiar with both of these forms of bodywork, but I was also very intrigued by chakra and energy work.

My desire to learn to do something with my hands took me to various "healing groups" in Berkeley, California, but I did not feel particularly inspired by them and feared that I would be flying back to Germany with "empty" hands. However, during my last weekend there, I took part in a healing workshop that would have a strong impact upon my future. Here I met a German woman who had just completed a Reiki course. When she told me about Reiki, I was impressed by her description of it: "You simply place your hands on your tummy, then it gets all quite hot and feels really good." Although this sounds all too simple, something about her convinced me that Reiki was too important to ignore and I became fascinated by its very simplicity and her conviction of its effectiveness. I felt overwhelmingly drawn to Reiki, even though I did not fully appreciate what it was and had no expectations about what it could do. It was as though I had been "struck" by something.

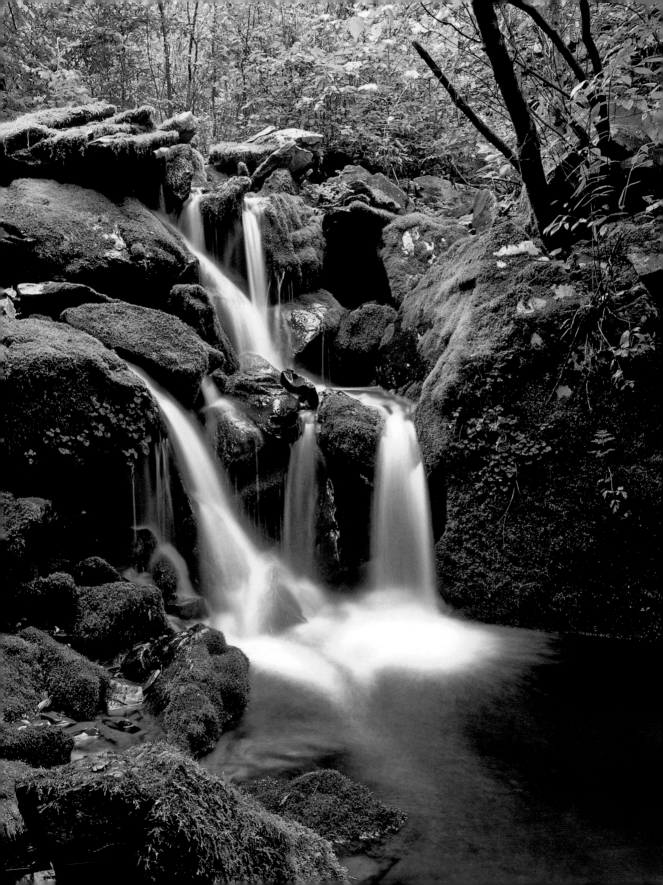

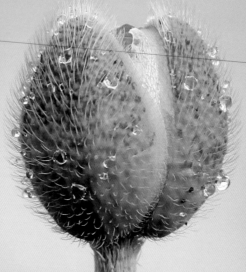

First Steps with Reiki

Because of the strength of my feeling for Reiki, I decided then and there to try to take a course in it before I flew home. I was lucky that the two Reiki Masters in San Francisco agreed to give me individual tuition in the First Degree (see pp. 46–9) on my last weekend in the United States. I received my energy attunements and learned the special hand positions. Now I was a Reiki channel. Still somewhat uncertain, I started tentatively to try out what I had learned so far. I distinctly remember giving a Reiki treatment to a woman in my guesthouse. This was an unforgettable moment for me because it was the first time I had ever experienced healing as a giver of hands-on treatment. The woman came to me with a bad headache, but felt better after her treatment – the pain in her head dissolved as my hands became hot and tingly. I could actually feel energy being drawn into her. We found Head Position Two (see p. 67) was particularly powerful.

> *"Reiki is such a gift, it has helped me so much, I am calmer, my intuition is sharper, and the world is so beautiful in my eyes. Reiki is the 'icing on the cake'."*
> JANE

The next day I flew back to Germany, where, at that time, Reiki was almost unknown. I had already become deeply involved with the technique and gave myself a self-treatment (see pp. 60–3) every day by treating my head, and the front and back of my body. In doing so, I contacted very deep levels in myself on physical, mental, emotional, and spiritual planes. Never before had I consciously fallen into states of such deep relaxation. I "saw" vivid colors and bright lights inside myself, but what impressed me most were the images and memories which put me in contact with past lives. The concept of reincarnation is a commonly accepted "truth" in Eastern religions and cultures whereby the physical body dies at the end of life but the soul is reborn, or reincarnated, repeatedly, into another body, until it reaches self-realization, or enlightenment.

I was overjoyed to have discovered something which could bring me closer to myself and for the next three months I treated myself with Reiki on a daily basis. I also exchanged Reiki treatments with a friend. We were impressed with our experiences and our relationship deepened.

My Second Degree

In Hamburg in November 1983, I was taught the Second Degree by Mary McFadyen, who had been taught by Hawayo Takata (who introduced Reiki to the West). Mary had come to Hamburg from the United States to teach Reiki. I remember very clearly how I felt sick and feverish the first night of the seminar, but that the following morning all the symptoms had disappeared. When I mentioned this to the group the next day, Mary said that this was quite a common experience among those learning Reiki and spoke of self-healing reactions which may occur during the seminar or after a Reiki treatment. She explained that because the energy in the body is strengthened by the initiation process, the vibratory rate of the body is amplified and adjusts to this "energy shift", which triggers the cleansing process (see p. 48). A sign that this initiation had worked, I thought.

Second Degree Effects

In the weeks immediately after the Second Degree, I noticed further changes in myself. I experienced what I describe as an "inner explosion". Energy had been set free in me. I felt fiery and strong. Only later did it become clear to me that Reiki had opened many new doors in my life. My intuition and self-confidence were enhanced as well as the intensity and effectiveness of my treatments. Some of my receivers (my clients) had deeply moving experiences during their treatments, coming into contact with old wounds and "hurts", which, once exposed to the light of day, could now be healed.

How I Used Reiki

At the start of a normal Reiki session, involving myself as the giver and my client as the receiver, I would use Mental Healing (see pp. 82–3) to work with more deeply seated emotional themes. This gave my work a new dimension. Through the Mental Healing I could come into contact with deeper levels of a person's unconscious. I was able to look for the cause

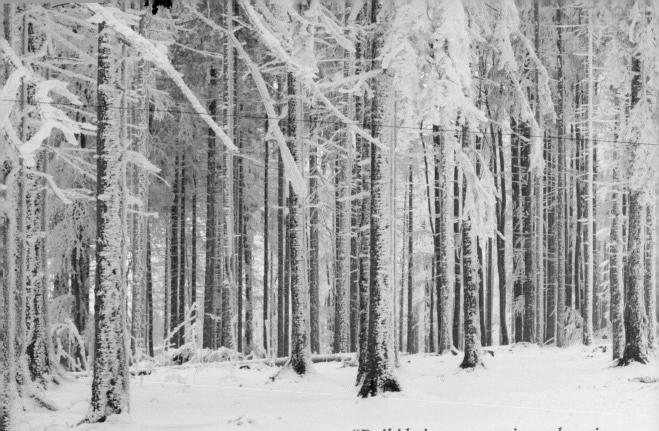

of a specific problem or disorder and I could also connect with the person's superconscious. I could ask for, be given, and recognize the right solutions during my treatments. Painful experiences from the past could be felt by the receiver and be relieved in a loving way. During this time I also treated myself daily with Mental Healing and continued to exchange Reiki treatments regularly with a friend. I felt myself to be in the flow of my own healing process as well as being able to help to heal others.

Other Areas of Self Growth

In the course of the years that followed I also became familiar with other methods of healing. These include psychic massage, Bach

"Reiki brings me again and again from the pressure of 'having to do' doing to the joy of being, non-doing, giving naturally."

KARIN

Flower Therapy, counselling, Aura Soma color therapy, and various forms of energy work and meditation techniques. Psychic massage therapy, in particular, had a great influence on my awareness of people's subtle body and energy fields. It is through this therapy method that I learned to do "psychic readings" of the chakras and the intuitive reception of images, emotions, and impressions which have shaped a person's life. With the help of massage, deep-seated feelings and energies are then released

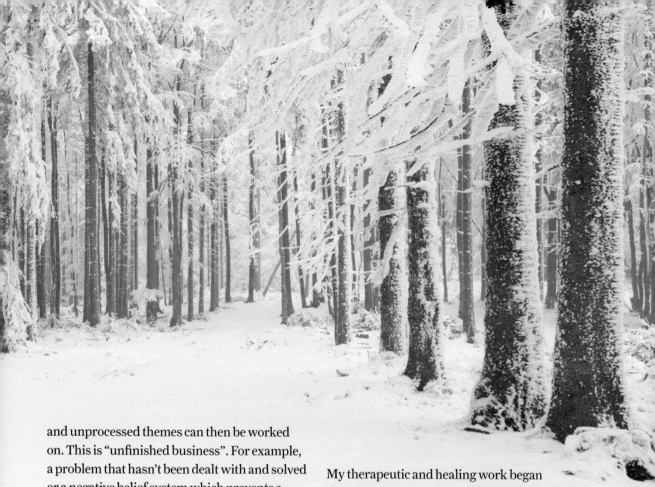

and unprocessed themes can then be worked on. This is "unfinished business". For example, a problem that hasn't been dealt with and solved or a negative belief system which prevents a person from living out his or her true potential. This type of body therapy touches people at deep levels of their being and allows them to see hidden aspects of their nature more clearly. I remember massaging a client's lower back and buttocks and receiving strong mental images of someone being beaten. I could feel tenseness and pain which turned into anger. When I asked my client how he felt, he said he could remember being beaten as a child.

Combining Reiki
Little by little Reiki brought me closer to myself and gradually helped increase my confidence.

My therapeutic and healing work began through Reiki and since 1983 I have combined it with massage and meditation. I find leading massage and meditation courses very enjoyable and my inner life is richer and more intense.

Looking back, I can now see that the different elements of my trainings gave my work with Reiki much more depth. In particular I found Bach Flower Therapy an effective method for the healing of discordant emotional conditions. The effects of the flowers are very quickly and clearly evident, particularly in animals and children: something that never fails to amaze me and which proves their power and effectiveness. I often recommend the flower therapy combined with Reiki, if, for example, a person is suffering from deep fears, depressions, exhaustion, mental strain, lack of self-confidence, despair, shock, and any other major emotional upsets.

About eight years after my first Reiki attunement, I felt a strong inner compulsion to take the Reiki Third (Master-Teacher) Degree (see pp. 56–7). I now knew that I was ready for it. Clients (my receivers) had also often asked whether they could learn Reiki from me, and I had always had to answer "no", since you cannot teach Reiki and attune others without becoming a Reiki Master. Now I knew that it was time for me to undertake my Reiki Master training.

My Reiki Lineage

In February 1992 I was trained as a Reiki Master-Teacher and initiated by Himani, who had herself received the Master Degree from Mary McFadyen. I felt integrated into the traditional Reiki lineage – Usui, Hayashi, Takata, McFadyen, Himani, and Tanmaya. The Reiki lineage is important because the essence of Reiki must remain pure in order to be powerful, and this can only happen if the original Symbols and original forms of teaching the technique remain untainted and intact. This, in turn, can only happen if the lineage is direct to the original source of Reiki (see p. 21).

After the Reiki Master initiation, which I received in India, I flew back to Germany and started to teach Reiki. The new experience of instructing and initiating others in Reiki made me feel very contented and fulfilled. I was conscious of the mission and responsibility of passing on the "essence" of Reiki to others.

In the course of teaching Reiki I also learned a great deal about myself. I came into very close contact with my spirituality and with my intuitive side. Through practicing Reiki so much, I felt pervaded and fortified by the Universal Life Energy. I was growing with Reiki and I greatly enjoyed teaching it to others, too.

The Move to England

In early 1993 I moved from Germany to England and I now hold most of my training courses there. I founded the South West School of Usui Reiki Healing in March 1995. For me, England is a very special country. The founder of Bach Flower Therapy, Dr Edward Bach, lived there and this is where he prepared his flower essences with garden and wayside flowers and blossoms. With his therapy he made a major contribution to the healing of discordant emotional conditions. I also love the mystical side of English nature and the countryside – it is still said by some that there are fairies and nature spirits in English gardens.

Since I have been living in England Reiki has taken a central role in my life. People who come to me to learn Reiki are characterized by an openness to the discovery of their own healing powers. Many arrive with a readiness and faith in the process of self-healing. Reiki is then the appropriate method or tool to make this possible. The First Degree seminars, in particular, deal mainly with the self-healing process and the recognition of one's own healing potential. In the Second Degree seminars we then enter deeper levels, dealing with the healing of emotional themes and sending healing energy from a distance. What has always continued to fascinate me about Reiki is its simple and direct effects. It is a healing method which passes through the hands, allowing energy, warmth, and love to flow into the receiver's body. This loving physical contact between two people has a healing effect, in itself. With Reiki enhancing this phenomenon the receiver then also receives the higher light energy which initiates and accelerates the healing process. This is what makes Reiki unique and differentiates it from the "loving touch" and other touch-healing techniques.

A Deep Connection

During a Reiki treatment, in which I am the giver, I feel deeply connected with the receiver, as if we are both immersed in a pool of silence and peace. I find Reiki to be a form of communication without words. My receivers often remark afterwards that they feel completely relaxed and more deeply connected with themselves as well.

The single most positive thing about giving or receiving Reiki is that it brings people closer together. It is a wonderful opportunity to deepen relationships with one another. It opens people up for others. It produces greater understanding between individuals and it breaks down barriers. Conflicts within the family or between friends can be resolved by giving and receiving Reiki together. Reiki can make life more enjoyable. In addition, anyone who is a channel for Reiki contributes to their own healing as well as to the healing of other people and the "whole". It is important to continue to make use of this power that unites all living things and to keep it flowing.

A New Culture

Today, Reiki meetings are held around the world, where Reiki channels can treat each other and compare notes. A new culture is being created by Reiki. Not just because it enhances our own lives, but it has a wider influence throughout society by changing people who influence the wider community.

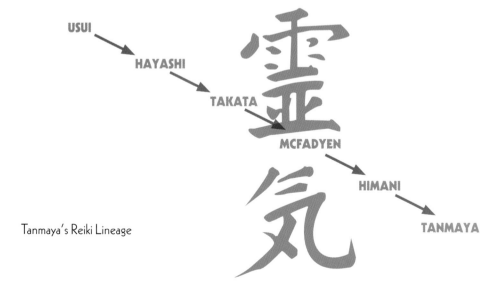

Tanmaya's Reiki Lineage

USUI → HAYASHI → TAKATA → MCFADYEN → HIMANI → TANMAYA

2. REIKI & ITS
MEANING

Reiki was rediscovered in the nineteenth century by a Japanese monk named Dr Mikao Usui. The tradition of Reiki is referred to in 2500-year-old writings in Sanskrit, the ancient Indian language. The Usui System of Natural Healing, named after Dr Usui, has been passed down by Reiki Masters since that time and is today practiced worldwide.

As humans we have Universal Life Energy all around us and within us. The Japanese word "rei-ki" consists of two syllables: "rei", which describes the cosmic, universal aspect of this energy and "ki", which means the fundamental life force flowing and pulsating in all living things. This life force energy is given to us at birth. We bring with us a certain amount of "ki" to life, and we use it up in the business of ordinary daily living. We then have to create a daily supply of new energy. When we are unable to make up for our energy consumption for a prolonged period, we may become physically or emotionally ill. If our supply of life force energy is very low and depleted, we suffer from physical, emotional and mental exhaustion, and tend to be much more irritable, bad-tempered, and depressed than usual.

We find different words for this fundamental force in all the different cultures and religions of the world. The Chinese know "ki" as "chi", Hindus say "prana", and Christians call it "light" and, in our modern Western language, we use the words "bioenergy" or "cosmic energy". In German, the words which come close to the meaning of "ki" are "Atem" – breath and "Leben" – life.

What is Reiki?

Reiki is a natural and simple healing method which allows you to absorb more life force energy. The Reiki method vitalizes your life force and balances the energies in your body. This natural healing energy flows in a powerful and concentrated form through the hands of the Reiki giver. The laying on of the hands directs the healing energy into the body of the receiver. The Reiki giver is used as a channel to conduct the Universal Life Energy. As a result, no personal energy is drawn or drained from the giver, who is simultaneously charged and strengthened.

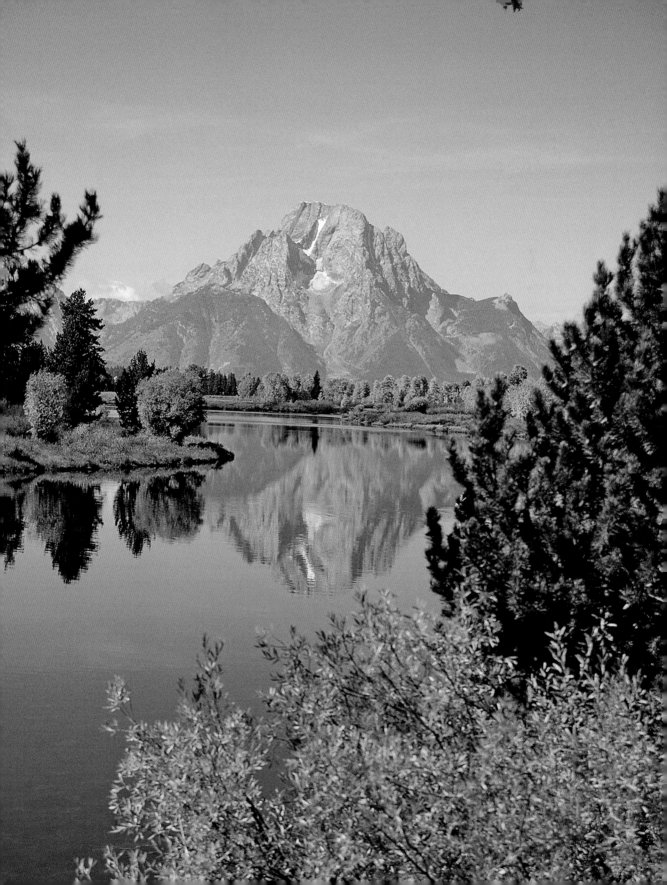

If you seek healing and are open and willing to let this healing power flow through you, then you can become a channel for the Reiki force. Once you are a channel then the ability to use Reiki remains within you for the rest of your life. This is a "truth" which is beyond proof in ordinary scientific terms.

Special Attunements

The key to Reiki is provided by "energy attunements", also known as "transmissions" or "initiations". These attunements differentiate Reiki from all other healing methods.

The special thing about these particular attunements is that they enable you to allow the Life Force Energy to flow through you more intensely. You receive one or more attunements depending on which Reiki Degree you are training in. The attunements are transmissions of energy which open your inner healing channel, allowing more

The Reiki symbols

The Japanese word "rei-ki" consists of two syllables: "rei", which describes the cosmic, universal aspect of this energy and "ki", which means the fundamental life force flowing and pulsating in all living things.

Rei – the cosmic, universal energy (top)

Ki – the fundamental life force (bottom)

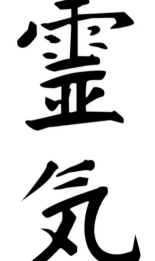

"I experienced a very deep sense of calm and peace. I felt that I had entered a very special place within me and felt certain that Reiki was a very welcome addition to my understanding of life."

MIKE

Universal Life Energy to flow through you. At each attunement, a kind of cleansing takes place on a physical, emotional, mental, and spiritual level. The attunements release blocks in you and toxins are set free.

When this happens you may experience self-healing reactions. This is a good sign and shows that your body first has to adjust to the higher life force energy vibration you are encountering (see pp. 38–40). The symptoms which may then appear are a part of the self-healing process (see also pp. 48).

Self-Healing

It is important to be aware that self-healing is the crucial first step in becoming a Reiki channel. Only when you take responsibility for your own healing are you in a position to support others in their own healing processes. Self-treatment leaves you feeling more relaxed, reducing stress and strengthening powers of resistance to illness. On a broader level, Reiki brings harmony and well-being into your life.

What does Reiki do?

Reiki usually helps healing of all kinds and relieves pains and acute symptoms quickly.

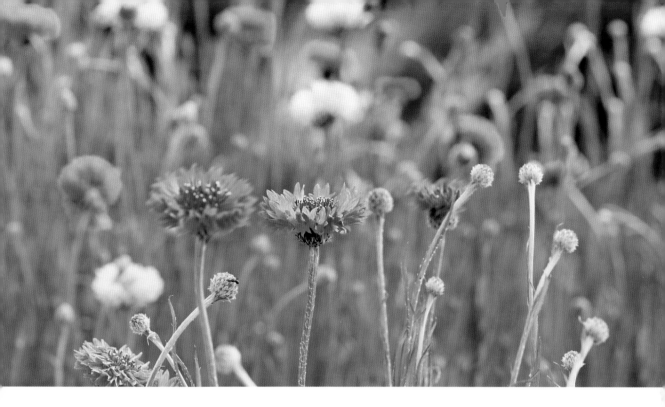

It also has a positive influence on spiritual growth. After a treatment, you may feel mentally much clearer about things and experience deep insights into particular questions or problems you are facing. Reiki can then help you to make the right changes and decisions in your life, if that is what you need or want to achieve.

Reiki affects each person differently, but it always acts wherever the receiver needs it most. However, there are common effects that everyone experiences. Energy used up in everyday life is replaced, so that when you feel exhausted or drained, the resulting imbalance, which may adversely affect you physically, emotionally, and mentally, can be put right.

If you suffer from stress, you may react with physical symptoms, such as headaches, stomach aches, frequent colds, kidney pains, and general digestive disorders. These symptoms are the expression of excessive negative stress, accompanied by an imbalance of the energy system. To relieve these symptoms your energy needs to be restored. For example, you may need to recharge a lower immune system, or a weak organ that is not functioning properly. Reiki can balance the energies in the body, helping you to let go and relax, so reducing stress. At the same time, it promotes the development of positive reactions to stressful situations. In other words, not only the symptoms but also the causes can be healed.

Reiki strengthens and harmonizes the immune system. We continually use up life force energy without replacing it. Reiki helps us to replenish and add to our energy and, in this way, helps to create a healthy body.

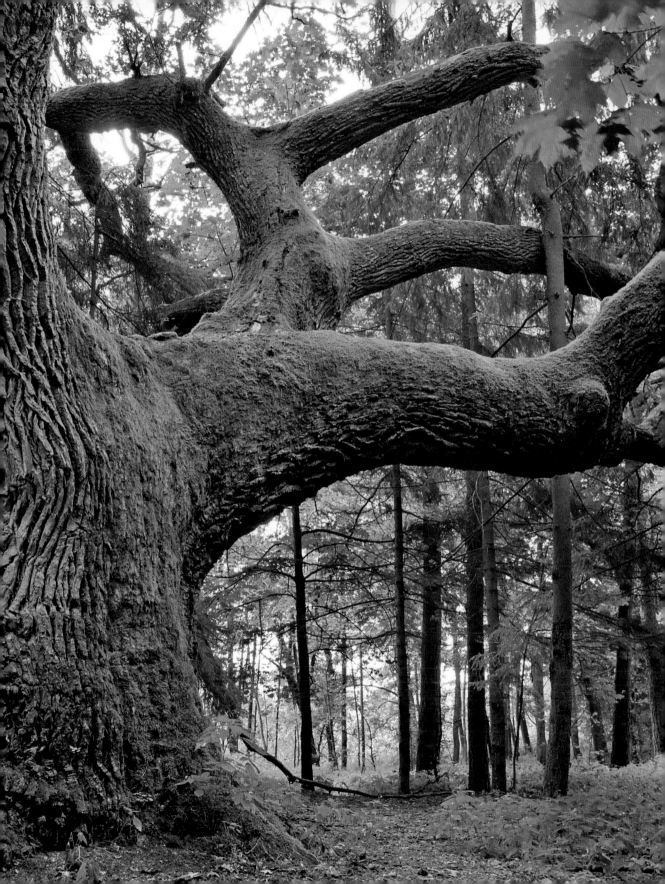

How Reiki Affects the Emotions

When you receive Reiki treatments or when you take part in a Reiki seminar your emotions may be profoundly affected. Emotional "blocks" are often released and you come into closer contact with feelings that you may have suppressed in the past – perhaps sadness or anger. It is important to accept these "negative" feelings. They are energies which transform themselves into creative forces as soon as you "own" them and give them attention and expression.

Reiki helps you to become more aware of your inner processes, both emotionally and mentally. During a Reiki treatment, the mind and the process of thinking are relaxed. You will often feel more clear-headed and might discover and dissolve negative beliefs about yourself and others that you have struggled with for many years.

Reiki supports you in your spiritual growth. People who open themselves to Reiki and practice it can get to know themselves better and can experience greater consciousness, intuition, and self-awareness. The most frequent experience which arises during a treatment is the feeling of peace, relaxation, and security.

"I feel that no matter what happens the energy is always available to be absorbed. Reiki means peace to me, life a continually flowing tap."
ZOE

Is Reiki Always Safe?

The purpose of Reiki is to supply the body with additional energy which it can use for healing itself. Reiki can also be used safely regardless of whatever illness the receiver is suffering from, but you should always seek the advice of a specialist doctor in addition to any Reiki you receive. Reiki makes no diagnoses and is intended to be used as a complementary healing method. In the case of acute disorders such as inflammations, influenza, colds, digestive disorders, gall or kidney stones, backaches, and headaches, Reiki often acts very quickly and directly by easing the pain and accelerating the healing process.

Reiki can also be applied directly as first aid (see pp. 96–7), as it helps to stop bleeding in open wounds and has a very calming influence on the nervous system, particularly when people are in shock after an accident. With Reiki, you can also provide relief from allergies, arthritis, and other chronic disorders.

As Reiki supports and complements other medical and natural healing techniques, you can combine it with other treatments, for example with allopathic or homeopathic treatments, body therapies, counselling and speech-therapy and other psychological treatments (see also p. 107). A Reiki healer is charged with energy and becomes a channel for Universal Life Energy. Reiki is a gift of the universe, available to us all.

THE EFFECTS OF
REIKI

In summary, Reiki is all-embracing in its effect. It involves your body, mind, and soul and then attempts to set all these aspects of your being into a harmonious balance. Your personal energy, as a giver, is not transmitted to the receiver during a treatment; you are merely a channel. If (without having attuned to Reiki) you try laying your hands on someone else, energy is still passed on, but at a much lower intensity than if you are attuned to Reiki. This is because Reiki is a highly powerful vibrating force, or light energy. to pupil. I'd like to share a brief explanation of it with you.

While the Universal Life Energy flows through you, as the giver, during a treatment, it is also fortifying and harmonizing you at the same time.

You may also experience Reiki as a force which brings you more closely into contact with yourself, opening you up and allowing you to be more loving with yourself and with others. It is a unifying force which brings you closer to a condition of oneness and connection with the "whole".

"Reiki has softened my outlook on life. It has made me realize that unknown things are real and important."

MIKE

What does Reiki do?

Reiki passes from giver (the Reiki channel) to receiver, working on many different levels. It brings all aspects of the receiver's being into harmonious balance, according to their individual needs and desires.

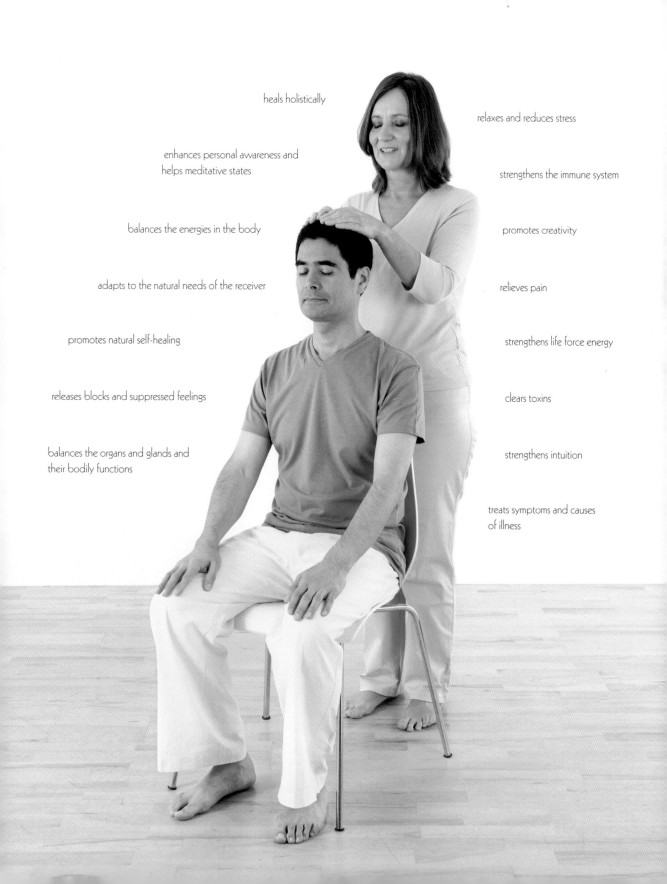

heals holistically

relaxes and reduces stress

enhances personal awareness and
helps meditative states

strengthens the immune system

balances the energies in the body

promotes creativity

adapts to the natural needs of the receiver

relieves pain

promotes natural self-healing

strengthens life force energy

releases blocks and suppressed feelings

clears toxins

balances the organs and glands and
their bodily functions

strengthens intuition

treats symptoms and causes
of illness

CHAKRAS &
THE ENDOCRINE SYSTEM

The Reiki treatment hand positions (see Chapter 5, pp. 58–81) correspond with the body's endocrine glandular system and the seven main chakras. The endocrine system regulates hormone balance and metabolism. On an energetic level, the endocrine glands correspond to the seven main chakras, or energy centers.

The word "chakra" comes from the Sanskrit, meaning "wheel". The clairvoyant can see the chakras as spinning energy spirals or colored chalices of light which differ in size and activity from one person to another. Our seven main chakras are seated in the human etheric body. They are connected to fine energy channels running along the spine. Without them the physical body could not exist. These energy centers collect subtle energy, transform it, and supply it to the body. Each chakra is "linked" with a certain organ and region of the body and has an influence on its function (see the chart on pp. 88–9).

The Endocrine System

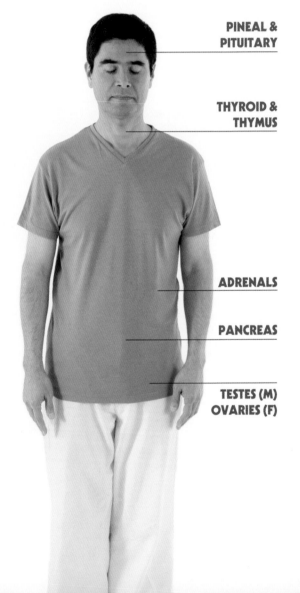

PINEAL & PITUITARY

THYROID & THYMUS

ADRENALS

PANCREAS

TESTES (M) OVARIES (F)

The endocrine and chakra systems

The hormones produced by the glands flow directly into the bloodstream or into the blood vessels of the organs, bringing vital energy into the body. The endocrine system supplies power to the chakras and, at the same time, leads the subtle energies of the chakras back into the body. Reiki operates through the interaction between chakras and endocrine glands and, in this way, involves the physical, energetic, and mental planes in the healing process. (See also pp. 86–7.)

The Chakras

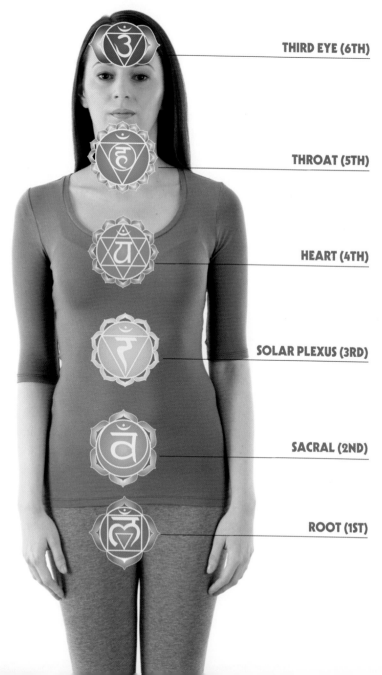

CROWN (7TH)

THIRD EYE (6TH)

THROAT (5TH)

HEART (4TH)

SOLAR PLEXUS (3RD)

SACRAL (2ND)

ROOT (1ST)

"How old you look and feel is directly related to the source of energy in the chakras. If you want to create an Ageless Body, you must 'will' energy into your body by concentrating on the endocrines."

CHRIS GRISCOM
THE AGELESS BODY

3. THE HISTORY OF
REIKI

The history of the Usui system of Reiki to date has always been handed down personally from Master to pupil. I'd like to share a brief explanation of it with you.

Dr Mikao Usui, the founder of Reiki, lived at the end of the nineteenth century and was the director and Christian priest of a small university in Kyoto, Japan. One day, some of his senior students asked him if he believed in the healing miracles of Christ and whether he was able to demonstrate such a healing. Dr Usui had no answer for this penetrating question. However, the incident led to great changes in his life. He gave up his position and started on a quest to study the healing methods of Christ. While he was searching he came across some material that greatly interested him in Buddhist scriptures.

Buddha, an enlightened master who lived around 600 BC, travelled as a monk through distant regions of India, and taught meditation and self-realization. In the years following his death, most of his followers were driven out of the country. As they fled they spread his teachings through Tibet, Nepal, Japan, China, and distant parts of Asia. Today, Buddhism is widespread in these Eastern countries. Usui was aware that Buddha had also possessed

the power of healing and so he searched for specific information on the methods Buddha used. Usui learned the ancient Indian language of Sanskrit and studied the original Buddhist writings in his quest for healing knowledge. In one of these ancient writings he found the Symbols and mantras which are the key to the Reiki system of healing. However, at that time Usui did not know how he should use the pictorial characters and names to bring about healing.

During his years of study, Usui spent a considerable time in a Buddhist monastery, where he became friends with the head abbot. On the abbot's advice, Usui embarked on a 21-day meditation and fast on a holy mountain near Kyoto. On the last day of his fast, he had a deep meditation experience. He saw a shining light in the sky which moved quickly towards him. This light struck him in the middle of his forehead (the Third Eye/Sixth Chakra) and he found himself to be in a state of extended consciousness. In this higher state Usui saw many small bubbles of rainbow-colored light

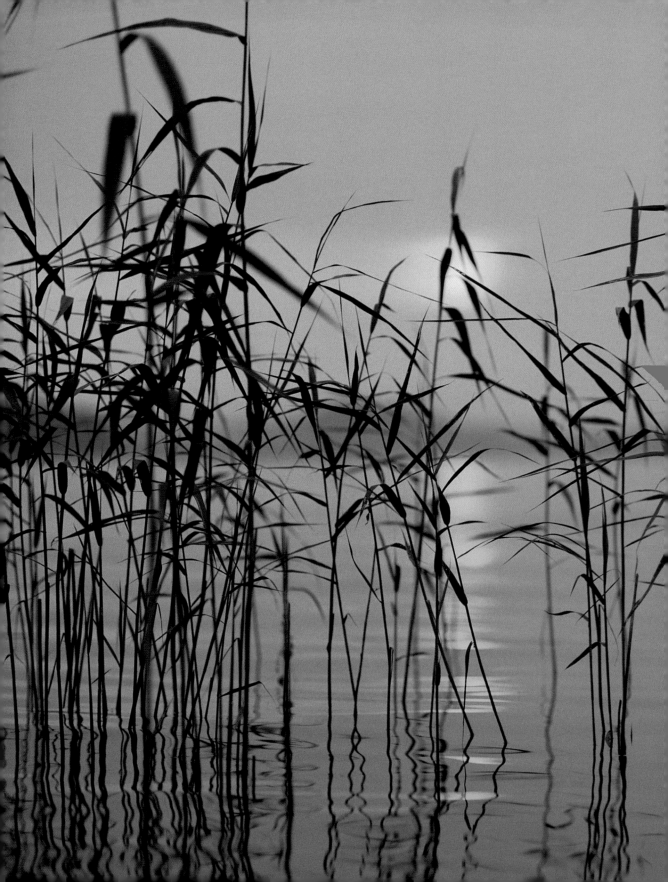

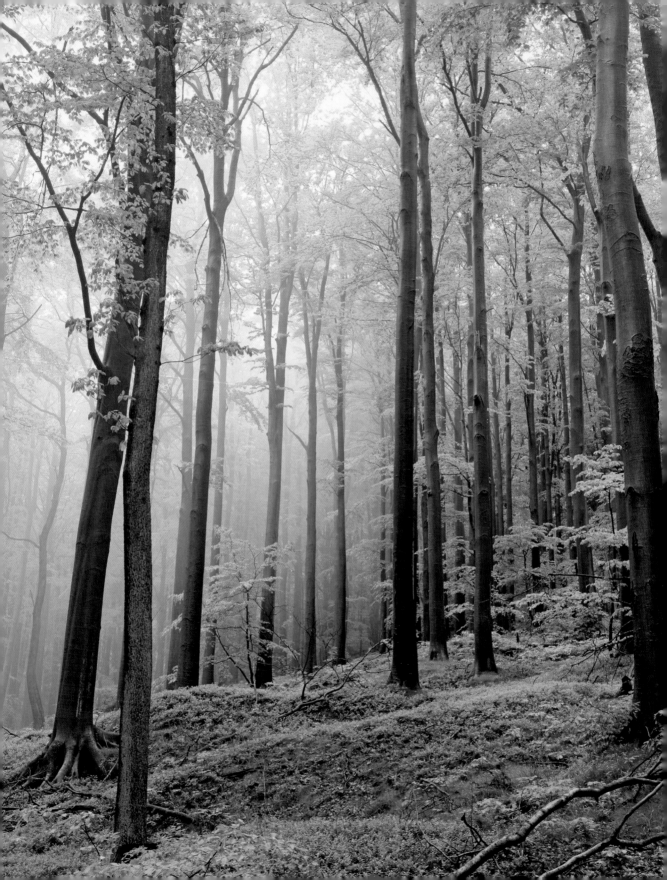

in front of him. Finally, a great white light appeared to him, in which, as if on a film screen, he recognized the familiar Symbols from the Sanskrit sutras, glowing in gold. Simultaneously, the application of the Symbols and mantras became clear to him and he felt charged with a powerful healing force. At the end of this incredible healing and enlightening experience, Usui began his descent from the holy mountain. In his haste, he stubbed a toe quite badly, causing it not only to throb but to bleed as well. When he held his hands around his foot, the bleeding immediately stopped and the pain vanished. This was his first experience of such extraordinary and rapid healing.

After Usui had spent a few weeks in the monastery of his friend, he decided to go to the slums of Kyoto in order to heal the sick. Through his seven years of experience in the slums, Usui came to recognize that, although he had healed the physical body of its symptoms of disease, he had not taught a new way of living. This prompted him to set out the Reiki rules for life (see p. 37). These principles, though laid down more than 100 years ago, are still of significance today.

Usui recognized that while many of the beggars he had treated had become healthy

"The healing that I was so in need of was beginning to happen. Something at last had opened up, had been cleared inside me."
DEBBIE

thanks to Reiki, they had not reintegrated themselves into society and were unable to handle their responsibilities. Usui realized how important the patient's own desire to be healthy was in the healing process. The sick person must ask for healing and he or she must really want it. Usui had offered his services free of charge in the slums. Now he saw how essential it is, when people receive healing, that they also give something in return. An energy exchange between healer and receiver is vital. On the basis of his experience in Kyoto, Usui now decided to travel in order to apply and to teach Reiki so that the way of thinking of the people would also be healed. A new phase began in his life.

A few years before his death, Dr Usui initiated a retired naval officer, Dr Chujiro Hayashi, in the Reiki method and declared him his successor. Dr Hayashi opened a private Reiki clinic in Tokyo. Here, Reiki practitioners were trained and patients treated. The Reiki healers worked in groups, often around the clock, and also made home visits. Dr Hayashi left documents and reports which showed that Reiki finds the cause of the physical symptoms, filling the body with the required energy and restoring it to wholeness.

Hawayo Takata, a young Japanese woman living in Hawaii, who was suffering from a number of serious disorders including a tumor, followed an inner call not to have an operation, but to seek healing in Japan. Through sheer coincidence, she heard of the Reiki clinic and went there for several months of treatment. As a result she became completely cured of her illnesses.

Takata became Hayashi's student and stayed with him there for a year. Then she returned to Hawaii, where she worked successfully as a healer.In 1938, she was initiated by Dr Hayashi as a Master of the Usui system. After Hayashi's death in 1941, Takata became his successor. She healed and taught for many years and, as far as is known, was the only Reiki Master until 1976. In the last years before her death, she began to train some of her students as Reiki Masters. By the time she died in 1980, she had initiated 22 Reiki Masters, among them her grand-daughter, Phyllis Lei Furumoto, who, in 1983, was recognized by the Reiki Alliance as a Grand Master of Reiki.

Through Takata and the Reiki teachers Furumoto had initiated, the art of Reiki healing became known in the Western world. Today, Reiki is known in every country in the world, and there are several thousand Reiki Masters. It is particularly widespread in Spain, Germany, Switzerland, England, Sweden, France, Italy, America, Canada, New Zealand, and Australia, and the continents of Asia and Africa are discovering Reiki. More exact information is not known since Reiki is spreading so rapidly. In the Second World War, Dr Hayashi's Reiki clinic was destroyed and Reiki was lost to Japan. Now, thanks to Western Reiki Masters, the Reiki art of healing is finding its way back to Japan.

Today there is a large number of directions and enormous variety within the Reiki healing method. Some Reiki Masters have formed themselves into organizations, while others work independently as free Reiki Masters and teachers. The traditional Reiki system still exists, representing the form and the content of the teaching in line with the original lineage of Usui, Hayashi, Takata, and Furumoto. Here we also find the original Symbols and mantras and the traditional initiation ritual. In addition, there are newly developed Reiki "branches", which also use the same universal energy for healing, but which may differ in the form and content of the teaching, the initiation rituals and the Symbols used.

Later Discoveries

There are numerous stories about Mikao Usui and the history of Reiki. A slightly different picture of Reiki's discovery and development came in the late 1990s from Japan, from two Reiki Masters, the German Master Arjava Petter and his Japanese wife Chetna Kobayashi. Their researches revealed that Usui had been a Buddhist, rather than a Christian, priest. It also became clear that Usui had passed his complete teachings on to 17 people, and not just to Chujiro Hayashi, as stated by Hawayo Takata. It became known that the teaching of Reiki had continued during and after the Second World War and that not all Reiki Masters had been killed in the war.

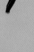

The Reiki principles

These are two forms of the Reiki principles. The version on the
right comes from the book by B. Müller and H. Günther,
A Complete Book of Reiki Healing. This is a modern, more
positive, wording of the original version, below, taken from
Mrs Takata's diary.

"Just for today, be free and happy.

Just for today, have joy.

Just for today, you are taken care of.

Live consciously in the moment.

Count your blessings with gratitude.

*Honor your parents, teachers
and elders.*

Earn your living honestly.

Love your neighbor as yourself.

Show gratitude to all living things."

"Just for today – thou shalt not anger.

Just for today – thou shalt not worry.

Be thankful for the many blessings.

Earn the living with honest labor.

Be kind to thy neighbors."

4. THE REIKI DEGREES

If you are a healthy person then Reiki is for relaxation, to relieve stress, and to restore personal energy. If you are unwell, or have a problem of some sort, whether this is on a physical, mental, emotional, or spiritual plane, Reiki may be the key you discover that allows you to take responsibility for your own healing. When you first use Reiki you open yourself to your own healing powers and become ready to accept the illness or the problem and to understand its message.

Reiki also gives you the courage to change the things in your life that you would like to change. Reiki gives you more power and energy to act and think responsibly in your life. Ask yourself: "Which old habits would I like to break?" Reiki can change your life. It can help you to find out more about yourself and bring you more self-awareness. It will speed up your physical, mental, and emotional healing and increase your spiritual growth.

If you give or receive a Reiki treatment you touch something deep within yourself. You could call it your "innermost being". Reiki is really an expression of love for yourself and for others and, in tune with the heart, it generates healing. Also, your intuition becomes sharper with Reiki. You gain access to the potential that is buried inside you. Each and every person is capable of self-healing and Reiki is a wonderful creative "tool" with which to access this ability.

The Reiki Symbols

In ancient times Tibetan monks recognized that our healing channels could be set to "vibrate", in order to transfer more energy. The Symbols and mantras they established are similar, and today they are used in Reiki to make these channels vibrate and to increase the vibrational frequency of the whole body.

A Symbol comprises a pictorial drawing and a name, also known as a "mantra". The drawing gives a visual representation of the symbol, while the name allows you to hear its sound and experience its vibration. In Reiki the mantra is repeated "inside", not out loud – you are working non-verbally on a thought wavelength to create vibration. This is similar in concept to telepathy.

Sound, such as music, is pure vibration, which puts something in motion. Music can influence you on different levels of your being.

You may enjoy some kinds of music, but dislike others. Your chakras, or energy centers, receive these vibrations. Classical music, for example, is usually soft and touches the heart center. Pop music is usually more strident and may reach or stimulate the Root (First) and Sacral (Second) Chakras. This music seems to want you to move your body. It draws certain types of people to it and supports a certain life style. Other kinds of music, for example, sitar music, stimulate the higher chakras, such as the Third Eye (Sixth) Chakra. Religious songs and mantra chanting also open the higher chakras and stimulate meditative experiences.

A Higher Vibration

Sound and mantras have the ability to vibrate certain chakras, depending on the vibratory level (or resonance) of the mantra and of the chakra. Through repetition of a mantra (for example, "OM") you can activate the upper energy centers.

In the attunement process of the First, Second, and Third Degree the Reiki Master uses Symbols and mantras to create a similar but much higher vibration than music is able to, and to channel Universal Life Energy. It is vitally important for everyone involved in Reiki to be aware that these Reiki Symbols and their mantras are confidential and are only passed on to students of the Second and Third Degree. They are therefore not published in this book.

We can say, however, that the First Symbol activates the general available energy. It is used wherever energy is lacking, for example in body treatment.

The Second Symbol adds a quality of harmony, peace, and balance to the etheric body (chakra system) and it is used especially for Mental Healing (see pp. 82–3).

The Third Symbol works at the mental level. It opens up intuition and strengthens the ability to "see". It is connected to the Third Eye (Sixth) Chakra and is used in Distant Healing, when energy and thoughts are sent to people who are physically absent.

The Fourth Symbol, or Master Symbol, strengthens the ability to open up to higher energies and to become a wide channel for them. The vibration of this Symbol is a very strong force and is used by the Reiki Master to channel higher energies during attunements. The Symbol can also be used for personal development and for meditation.

The Importance of Attunement

To become a Reiki "channel" you must first establish an "attunement" to the Reiki power.

"Reiki is a beautiful gift to others and to myself. The energy attunements have opened new gateways and brought magnificent change into my life on different levels."
GEORGE

How attunement is experienced

Everyone experiences Reiki in their own way. Each person brings their own past into it and may experience attunement differently to others. For some it is like an initial ignition. Energy is activated gently but powerfully, and the body is stimulated to "vibrate". Attunement starts at the point you have reached in your spiritual development, so that how much energy you can absorb and integrate depends on your own development. If you are already experienced in esoteric matters, you will feel transmitted vibration and be energetically charged with a correspondingly higher frequency. This energy stays with you for life.

"It was like being reconnected to the source and I felt more complete. There was a tremendous sense of relief..."
HELENE

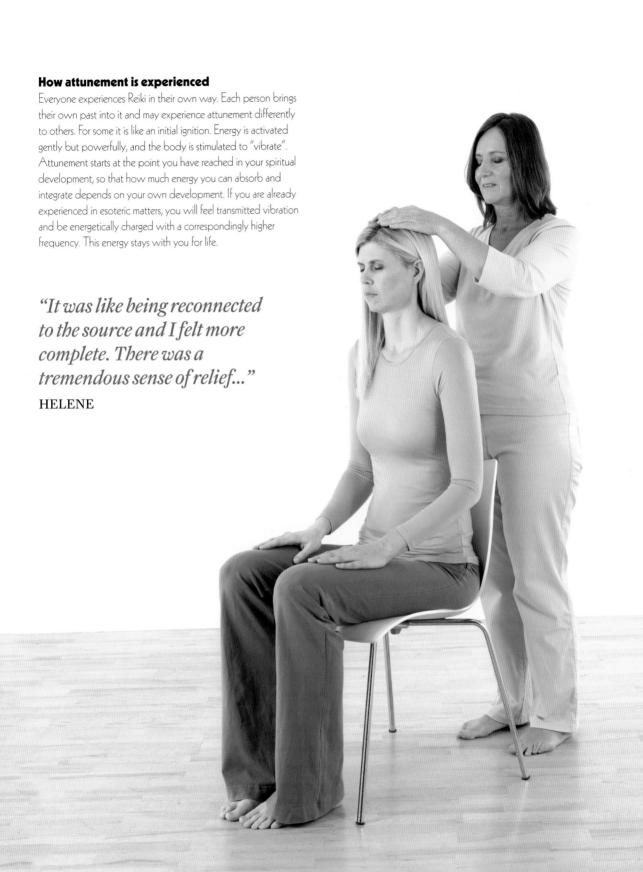

*"During and after
the attunement I felt a
tremendous energy release
at the center of my heart and
I felt very vulnerable. I think
I have grown a lot softer and
seek not to judge so much..."*

HELENE

This really means reconnecting with
and accessing the Universal Life Energy.
Attunement is the special key to the Reiki
system, and is what makes it a unique
healing method that is quite different from
all other hands-on healing techniques.
Attunement is also commonly referred
to as "energy transmission" or alternatively
as "initiation".

Using an ancient Tibetan technique, the
Reiki Master transmits energy to the students.
These attunements open the inner healing
channel. The attunement process usually takes
the form of a simple ceremony in which the
Reiki Master attunes each person individually
into the Reiki healing method. The Master uses
the confidential Reiki Symbols and mantras
(see pp. 38–40 for theory) to amplify the flow
of energy to the student.

The energy enters your body through the
top of your head, and flows through the upper
energy centers, known as chakras. It continues
down your arms, and leaves your body by
radiating from your hands. This energy is
now available to be used for healing yourself and others.

Common Perceptions

Although people experience the attunement
process differently, in their own way, there are
some common perceptions. For example, many
students experience a stronger energy flow
in the body which often manifests itself as a
pleasant wave-like flow and expansive feeling
of warmth across the whole of the body. Others
see a bright white light or a whole variety of
vivid colors in their mind's eye.

Many Reiki initiates experience a deeper
emotional and spiritual encounter with
themselves. A space of peace, quiet, and
meditation opens up which engulfs the
Reiki Master and student together.

Opening your Channel

Regardless of what you experience during
the attunement process – and even if you feel
you have experienced nothing – your inner
healing channel is opened. For those who are
"open" to Reiki, this process is automatic. You
do not need to "make" it happen. However, the
more "present" you are during the attunement
process and the more you abandon yourself to
it, the more energy will be absorbed. Once you
have become a Reiki channel you will retain this
ability for the rest of your life. Even after a break
of several years you can immediately use the
Reiki power again.

Using your Channel

While you will always be able to tap into the
power Reiki provides once you have been
initiated, it is important to use this healing
channel as often as possible. Imagine a water
pipe that is used regularly through which the

water runs clear and clean. However, if this pipe is used only occasionally, contaminants may accumulate and impede water flow. The water will also be less pure. This is similar to what can happen to your healing channel. The more often you use it the more easily and strongly the Reiki energy will flow through it. After the First Degree try to give yourself one daily treatment for a minimum of three weeks to three months. After that treat yourself as often as you wish to.

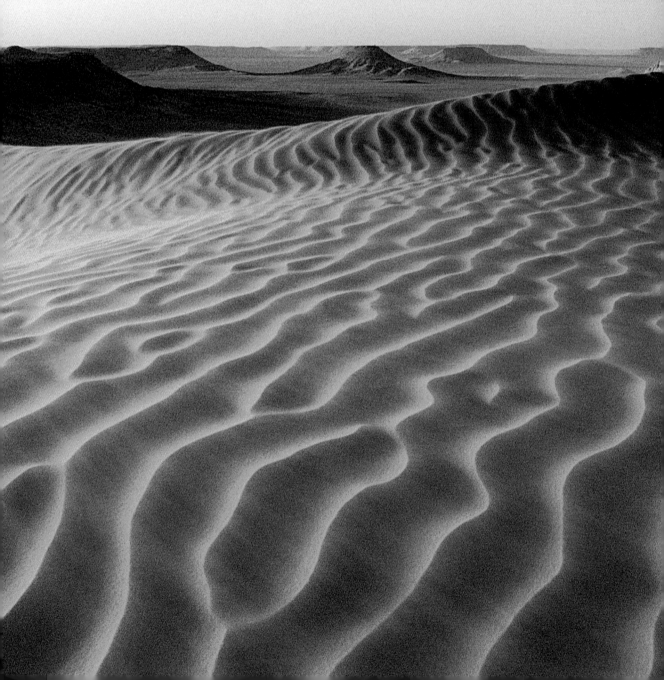

BREATHING
EXERCISE

If you want to experience a "taster" of Reiki before actually committing yourself to attunement, try this exercise. The exercise will have the same relaxing effects as Reiki, but without the added power and impact provided by the Universal Life Energy through attunement.

"I find that Reiki restores me if I'm tired or distressed in any way. My intuition, also, is greatly enhanced."

JIM

2. Now put your hands on your body wherever you feel drawn to or where you feel tension. Use your intuition to locate the spot in your body that will benefit from relaxation the most.

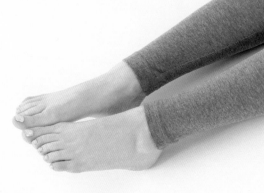

1. Make yourself comfortable, either sitting down or lying on your back, and close your eyes. Pay attention to your breath and follow its rhythm. Notice how it flows in and out.

3. Now direct your breath consciously and repeatedly to this place. Imagine that your breath is the Universal Life Energy which flows through you. Let it collect and expand under your hands. Notice how a feeling of relaxation and peace gradually spreads from that place beneath your hands throughout your entire body.

4. After a short while (about five minutes) place your hands on another part of your body. Once again, breathe into your hands during the whole exercise. You may find that your breath changes in some positions as the body stores memories and experiences which can now be awakened. It is not necessary to consciously probe feelings or initiate stronger breathing. Just allow yourself to let go and to plunge into this feeling of flowing.

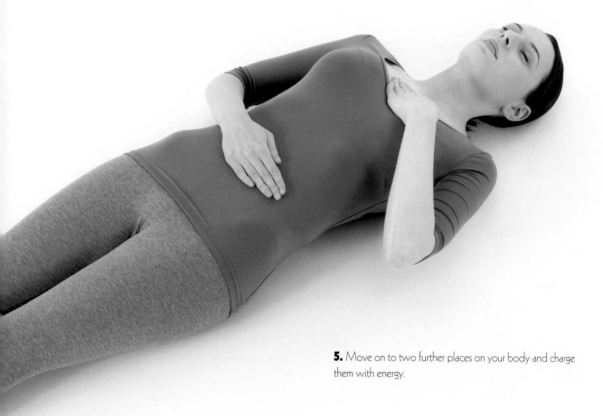

5. Move on to two further places on your body and charge them with energy.

6. Slowly open your eyes, stretch yourself, and return to your normal daytime consciousness. You will feel more relaxed, calmer, and more centered.

THE FIRST
DEGREE

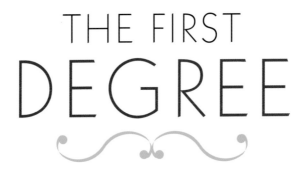

Traditionally, training in the Reiki methods spans three Degrees, which are self-contained. You progress from one degree to the next according to your own rate of personal experience and inner growth. There are no special conditions or equipment required to learn and practice Reiki, but people who want to be open to Reiki tend to have a natural readiness and ability to receive it. People of any age (including children) can acquire the skill of Reiki. It is not uncommon for whole families to learn it. Among friends or within a family Reiki offers a very positive opportunity to spend time together in a warm and secure atmosphere.

First Degree Reiki is a basic course which is usually held as a weekend seminar. During a two-day period you learn something about the history of Reiki and the hand positions for treatment.

Attunement

Each First Degree participant is given four attunements, also called "energy transmissions", during which he or she receives a transfer or reactivation of Universal Life Energy. The attunements adjusts the vibrations of the Reiki student to the higher vibration of the Reiki power, so that more energy can flow through the body.

The attunements increase the vibration frequency of the four upper chakras – the Fourth (Heart), Fifth (Throat), Sixth (Third Eye), and Seventh (Crown) Chakras. The attunements to the First Degree mainly open the physical body so that you can take in more Universal Life Energy and let more of it flow through you. During the seminar the Reiki Master gives individual attunements. He or she also teaches the hand positions for treating the whole body. How the hand positions affect particular organs and body parts is also explained. You also learn hand positions for treating certain illnesses and for First Aid (see pp. 96–7).

"The process of becoming a Reiki channel has been an eye-opener for me – especially the First Degree."
HANNAH

"I felt very good and experienced 100 percent energy for at least three weeks after my attunement. I feel Reiki has strengthened everything. It has opened my intuition on a deeper level."

SANDRA

The attunement process

During the process known as attunement, the Universal Life Energy is transferred and activated via four attunements, or "energy transmissions".

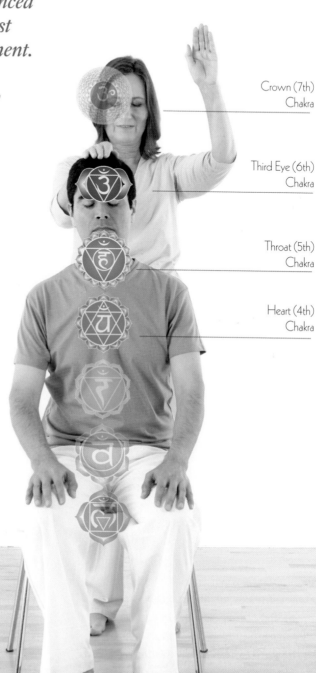

Crown (7th)
Chakra

Third Eye (6th)
Chakra

Throat (5th)
Chakra

Heart (4th)
Chakra

After the First Degree

Following the First Degree attunements Reiki energy flows through your hands and you can now give Reiki to yourself and to others. You may notice how a healing warmth radiates from your hands which may be accompanied by a tingling or pulsating in them. The Universal Life Energy always flows according to the requirements of the receiver, who absorbs only the amount of energy he or she needs. During treatments that you give you feel very distinctly that you are a channel: no energy is taken away from you; instead it passes through you. After giving Reiki you may also feel recharged and refreshed.

Self-Healing and Cleansing Reactions

You may notice that you develop certain physical symptoms during the weekend seminar and the days after the attunement. These reactions are a good sign because they show that the healing process is active within you. As in homeopathy, a "crisis" is reached so that the toxic energy can leave the body completely (see below). Drinking plenty of water during the seminar is good for helping this cleansing process.

Each attunement triggers a form of cleansing, as the energy system first needs to adjust to the higher vibration. If there are any blockages – physical, mental, emotional, or spiritual – Reiki will bring out what is hidden below the surface in order to provide healing and balance. If you feel suppressed experiences returning to the surface, this is often the right time to acknowledge and deal with them, although this may not always

be convenient. You may be confronted with feelings that you have been holding back, or you may experience strong physical exhaustion. The opposite also occurs: you may feel totally revitalized and far more lively than usual. Some people feel a cold coming on, which then subsides within a few hours. Others have a headache or experience "pins and needles" in their heads. These self-healing responses tend to subside in the course of the seminar, often within a few hours or a day at most. These strong reactions show that the healing process is in progress.

Daily Treatment

It is a good idea to work on yourself for some time after a First Degree Reiki seminar. Daily self-treatment strengthens your health and your life force energy is recharged with each session. Furthermore, your individual experiences in dealing with Reiki are very helpful to better understand the reactions of other people. You should aim first of all to love and heal yourself because you can only give to others what you are prepared to give to yourself.

"I experienced Reiki as helping me to travel down my new road by providing energy and fresh insight, and helping me to let go of old, less healthy, ways of being."

SAM

The more frequently you use Reiki, the stronger the energy flow inside you will be. Simply make it a habit to give yourself Reiki at certain times of the day. For example, in the morning, when you wake up, take twenty or thirty minutes to treat your head (see pp. 60–1) and the front of your body (see p. 62), or put your hands on whichever part of the body you feel needs attention. During the day, at odd moments, such as when you are making a phone call, watching television, or when you are waiting for something or making a journey, Reiki will have a beneficial effect and will refresh you. In the afternoon if you are tired and need a little break, try treating your Solar Plexus (Third) Chakra with the Quick Energizer (see p. 50). If you have difficulty getting to sleep, the Sleep Help treatment can also be very helpful (see p. 51).

Even if you have not yet been attuned to Reiki you can still use the Quick Energizer and the Sleep Help position, which provide beneficial, though weaker, energy. If you are already a Reiki channel your energy level will be charged with a higher vibration.

"The First Degree gave me great confidence, and a place in the world I had not known before."
DON

A Word of Caution

The contents and techniques of the First Degree seminar are in and of themselves complete, and enable you to treat yourself and others. But it is important to be aware that Reiki is not a substitute for treatment by a doctor, or for orthodox medication. Reiki will, however, support any form of therapy and the natural healing process. It is therefore ideal for complementing the work of nurses, doctors, midwives, care assistants for the elderly, massage therapists, shiatsu practitioners, aromatherapists, reflexologists, acupuncturists, and breathing therapists, as well as all non-medical practitioners. If you are attuned in Reiki, the Universal Life Energy automatically contributes to any hands-on treatment as soon as there is physical contact.

"I feel very privileged to have been given this gift and to be able to share the experience of Reiki with others both in giving and receiving."
HELENE

QUICK ENERGIZER

This simple Reiki exercise is a good way of replenishing depleted energy during the day. A few minutes spent will be rewarded with feelings of renewed energy and refreshment.

1. Find a comfortable place to sit or lie down and relax.

2. Put one hand over your Solar Plexus (Third) Chakra.

3. Place the other hand directly underneath, touching your stomach.

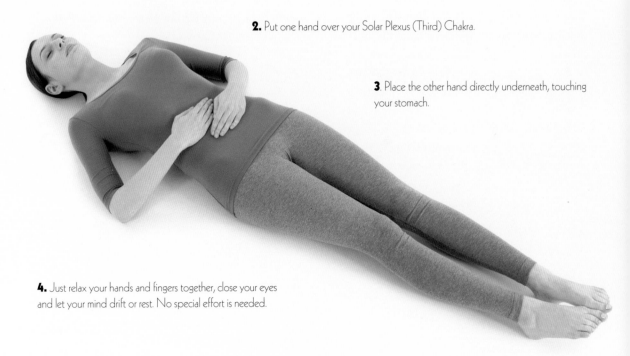

4. Just relax your hands and fingers together, close your eyes and let your mind drift or rest. No special effort is needed.

5. Stay in this position for 10 to 15 minutes. Afterwards you will feel rejuvenated and refreshed with vital energy.

SLEEP HELP

If you cannot get to sleep at night for any reason, this position will encourage the deep relaxation you need in order to fall asleep without any problems.

1. Get comfortable in your normal sleeping position, either lying on your back or side.

2. Now place one hand on your forehead and the other on your stomach. Notice your stomach rising and falling while you breathe.

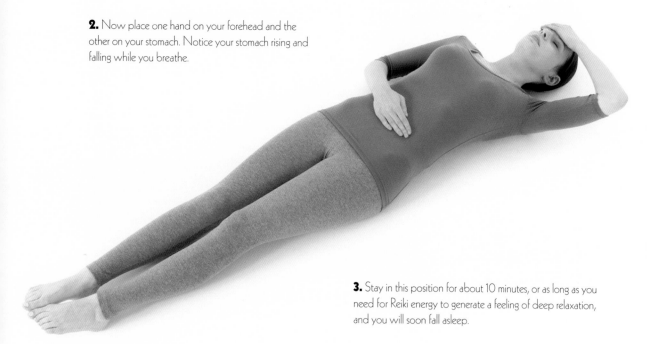

3. Stay in this position for about 10 minutes, or as long as you need for Reiki energy to generate a feeling of deep relaxation, and you will soon fall asleep.

THE SECOND
DEGREE

If, having been attuned to the First Degree, after some weeks or months you feel you have gathered experience with Reiki and would like to learn more to make your treatment deeper and more meaningful, then now is the right time to learn the Second Degree.

In Japanese this Degree is called "Oku Den", meaning a more thorough exploration of the Self – or "deeper knowledge". Think carefully about whether the right time has come for you to receive the Second Degree, as it is a mistake to rush into it – it sets much in motion on all levels. It has a particular effect on the etheric body (chakra system) and your intuition and healing ability is greatly expanded. Allow one to three months between the First and Second Degree attunements to process the energetically triggered inner processes completely.

Paula Horan has described a twenty-one-day cleansing process (see also pp. 24 and 48) after each Degree. As the attunements increase the vibrational frequency of the physical and etheric body (chakra system) they also bring any negative energies within to the surface to be released. Usually the Reiki power takes about three days to modify each chakra, so the complete process lasts twenty-one days. Although the Reiki channel is opened between

the Heart (Fourth) and the Crown (Seventh) Chakras, the lower chakras – Root (First) to Solar Plexus (Third) are equally important and are also adjusted to the Reiki power during a cleansing period.

The Second Degree gives you a technique to help you to use energy in non-physical dimensions. You learn to send healing energy across a distance, referred to as Distant Healing. This is the transmission of light energy to a recipient a distance away; similar, in some ways, to ordinary radio signals. Furthermore, you learn a special method for handling any deeply emotional and mental problems. Mental Healing, as it is called, allows you to contact the subconscious, and the superconscious, or the Higher Self, and to bring about healing in the receiver via the spirit. This is used to address problems such as sleeplessness, addictions, depression, or nervousness. You can also give Mental Healing to yourself, perhaps to transform usual behavioral patterns into more positive ones. In this Degree a further attunement greatly strengthens your healing powers. This primarily stimulates the Third Eye (Sixth) Chakra. It operates like a sensitive antenna. Second Degree Reiki works on the development of your intuitive powers and you are able to open yourself more easily to the deeper meaning of messages.

You are also given the confidential Reiki Symbols and the corresponding mantras (see pp. 38–40 for theory). They increase your energy and generate a higher light vibration within you. These are the same Symbols as those "seen"

by Dr Usui (see p. 35) and are only meant for those attuned to the Second Degree. Using these Symbols carries great responsibility. Thus each Reiki Master judges potential participants in a Second Degree seminar and decides whether they are responsible enough to work with the Symbols. Not everyone can cope with such responsibility – for example, those who suffer from mental disturbance. Most people ask to learn the degree only when they feel ready and then still must be judged as capable of taking it on.

Attunement

The Second Degree Reiki attunement increases the energy in the chakras still further. The three Reiki Symbols are also activated now. This attunement sharpens the intuition and the imagination, needed for Distant and Mental Healing. The "quantum leap" in the increase of the vibration frequency is several times stronger on the Second Degree than for the attunement to the First Degree. This is one of the basic "truths" of Reiki – something which has to be experienced to be properly understood.

DISTANT HEALING
VISUALIZATION

This is an exercise which you can use to send Reiki or certain loving and healing thoughts across a distance. During the time of remote contact the golden light has a protective function and means that you cannot be energetically disturbed by another possible source (perhaps someone in your life who is making demands on you at the moment). (See also pp. 84–5.)

N.B. Distant Healing must never be sent to anyone undergoing an operation, since it can undermine the effects of the anesthetic. However, it can be used safely both in preparation for the operation and to assist natural healing processes afterwards. This applies to people and animals.

1. Imagine that you are full of a golden light that charges your whole body and radiates from it. This light encases your body like a protective shell.

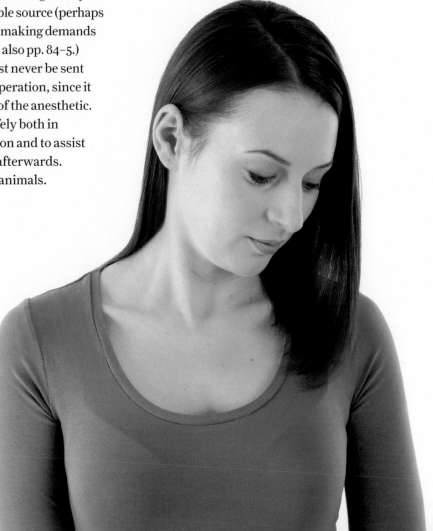

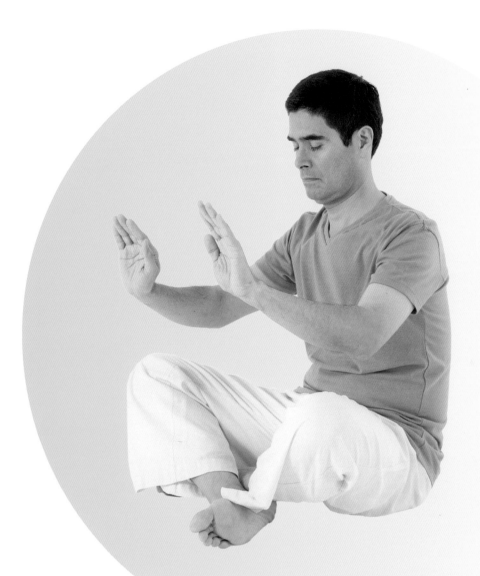

2. Now "feel" or "see" the person to whom you want to send some healing. If you are attuned to the Second Degree, you can use the Symbols for remote healing at this point (see pp. 38–40 for the theory). Once the person "appears", he or she is also included in this light.

3. Now send the light energy from the palms of your hands to the person to be treated through visualization. Direct the palms of your hands toward the visualized person. Imagine two laser-like beams of light flowing as healing energy from your palms into the body of the receiver. You can also imagine sending loving and healing thoughts to that person.

4. At the end of the exercise imagine the light that encompassed both of you slowly dispersing.

THE THIRD (MASTER)
DEGREE

When you decide to follow the path of the Reiki Master and take the Third (Master) Degree you must feel a vocation to give and receive healing. You may have the urge to find out more about yourself and to use this experience to help others to discover and to love themselves. When you are acquiring the Third (Master) Degree you make a commitment to practice, teach, and ultimately, to live, Reiki. Once you have practiced the First and Second Degree for between one and three years, and you have gathered sufficient experience with Reiki, then this is the time to register for the Third (Master) Degree.

The training for this degree is a process of growing into the mysteries and depths of the healing processes with Reiki, which takes dedication and experience. Energy-wise the Third Degree requires time and commitment if you are to process the many reactions which Reiki triggers in you at this level.

If you are interested in studying for this Degree, ask yourself: "Why do I wish to become a Reiki Master? Do I feel mature enough to carry this responsibility? Do I have enough experience with Reiki?" The Third Degree demands high spiritual maturity. It is a major life commitment, lifting your energy and consciousness to a far higher level than before. If you become a Master, Reiki interacts with all aspects of your life. It cannot be "compartmentalized", but is integral to everything you do. You have to "live" Reiki.

Not everyone can do this. If you want to make Reiki an important part of your life, then the path to the Reiki Master is for you. This most intense attunement starts a deep-reaching development and enables substantial personal growth on all levels. You have to investigate and challenge old thought and behavioral structures and you may have to reject and replace them. As a Reiki Master you will come to recognize that you are master of your life. Until the beginning of 1988 there were just two Reiki Masters who were authorized by Hawayo Takata to initiate Reiki students in the Third (Master) Degree. These were the Reiki Masters Barbara Weber-Ray and the grand-daughter of Hawayo Takata, Phyllis Lei Furumoto. In early 1988, the Grand Master Furumoto granted authorization for all Reiki Masters with a minimum of three years of active practice to initiate others in the Third (Master) Degree. This recommendation of the International Reiki Alliance is today not observed by all practicing Reiki Masters. Over the last 5–10 years many Masters have divided the Third Degree into Master and Master-Teacher. The Master Degree (also titled Master-Practitioner) comprises of receiving the Master symbol and its usage in daily life. The Master-Teacher Degree makes you a qualified Master-Teacher, where you learn the initiation process and how to pass on the knowledge of Reiki to others.

Attunement

The training program for a Reiki Master is individually tailored and should take place over a period of time. I consider it important that every aspiring Reiki Master first assists in the First and Second degree seminars. Here, Reiki students refresh their knowledge, for example perfecting mastery of the Symbols and mantras. They also learn the methods of instruction and again clarify the sequence of the seminar. As you contemplate becoming a Reiki Master you should feel confident in your ability to teach Reiki to others, since that is your main focus as a Master. Important in the training is the complex process of stimulated energy transmission with all the associated Symbols. In the last part of the training, the student receives initiation in the Master Symbol, the fourth Reiki Symbol. From this point on students are capable of activating the higher vibration of the Fourth Symbol and of feeling it within themselves. They can direct the force of this Symbol for personal growth and towards their work with others. In this way, Reiki becomes a vehicle on the path to personal perfection.

5. THE REIKI TREATMENTS

Reiki allows you to experience a higher energy vibration. When you give or receive Reiki, you reach a state of enhanced equilibrium and well-being. You reconnect to the source of Universal Life Energy and strengthen your self-healing powers, assuming responsibility for your own good health. You recognize this energy flowing through you, nourishing you and keeping you alive. This energy is the power that lives and acts in all created matter.

Before each treatment, spend time in quiet contemplation or meditation. This creates a loving atmosphere which encourages relaxing and letting go, both in you, the giver, and your receiver. You, the giver, are only a channel, and have no influence on the result of the treatment.

The amount of energy absorbed by the receiver always depends on his or her needs, though it may take time for the body to open up to receive this healing energy. This differs from person to person. A receiver does not need to open to Reiki because the body absorbs whatever Reiki energy it needs automatically.

Lay your slightly cupped hands, fingers closed and relaxed, on the receiver without exerting pressure, following his or her body shape. Your hands may become hot and tingle or throb. This is natural, reassuring you that Reiki is flowing. When you touch places which feel hot or cold, you have found the source of a problem: a chronic or acute disorder may well exist there. Keep your hands on until you sense that energy flow has normalized. Use your intuition to judge when this is.

When Reiki is Useful
Use Reiki to help and to heal; but never as a substitute for medical care or medication. It is capable of reinforcing every therapy and activates your own self-healing powers.

Reiki is particularly helpful before and after an operation, as it produces harmony and calms the receiver. Reiki also accelerates the healing process, causing operation incisions to heal more quickly and more satisfactorily. This is because the Reiki energy is intense and the body draws in what it needs.

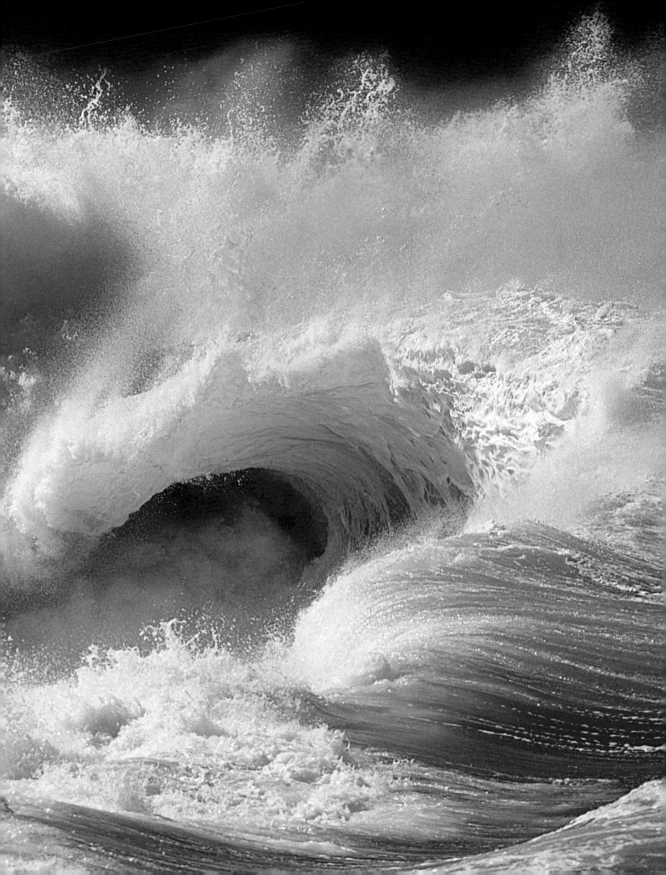

SELF-TREATMENT THE HEAD

You can use Reiki self-treatment simply and effectively on yourself at all times; it requires no extra equipment or props. Give yourself a full treatment whenever you get the chance. Use the same positions as you would use when treating someone else. The following pages show the self-treatment sequence, which you can carry out either sitting or lying down. The sequence takes between forty-five minutes and one hour to complete. Remain in each position for about three to five minutes. Lay your hands gently on the different body positions, starting with the head, working down the front of the body, and ending by treating the back. If you have pains or definite problem areas, let your hands rest on the problem area. Simply be creative with your hands. Let yourself be led by them and follow your intuition.

(See p. 138 for a Guided Self-Treatment CD.)

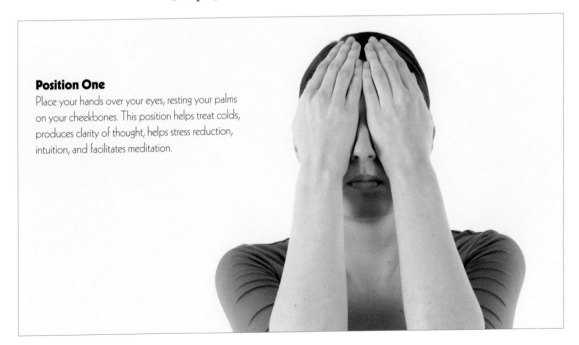

Position One

Place your hands over your eyes, resting your palms on your cheekbones. This position helps treat colds, produces clarity of thought, helps stress reduction, intuition, and facilitates meditation.

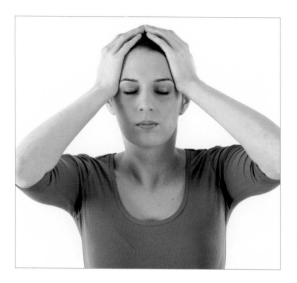

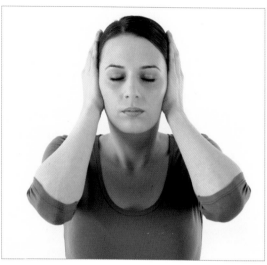

Position Two

Place your hands on both sides of your head, above your ears, touching the temples. This position harmonizes the two sides of the brain, improves memory and enjoyment of life, and is helpful for depressions and headaches.

Position Three

Place your hands on both sides of the head, covering the ears. This position is very comforting and affects the whole body. It is helpful for earache and eases the symptoms of colds and flu.

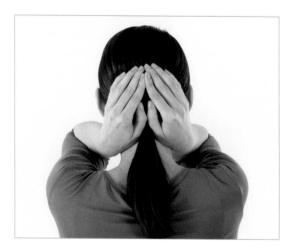

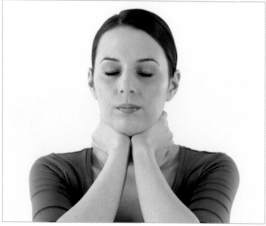

Position Four

Place your hands on the back of your head, holding it like a ball. This position eases sleep disorders, conveys a sense of security, promotes intuition, helps headaches, relieves fears, and depression, and calms the mind and the emotions.

Position Five

Place your hands around your throat, wrists touching in the center. This position harmonizes blood pressure and metabolism, helps neck pains and hoarseness, and promotes self-expression.

TREATING YOUR FRONT

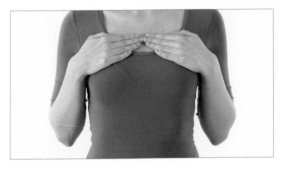

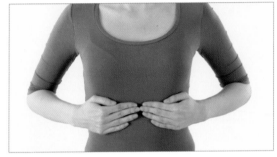

Position One

Place your hands on the left and right sides of your upper chest, fingers touching just below the collarbone. This position strengthens the immune system, regulates heart and blood pressure, stimulates lymph circulation, increases the capacity for love, enjoyment of life, transforms negativity.

Position Two

Place your hands over the lower rib cage above the waist, fingers touching. This position regulates the digestion, gives energy, promotes relaxation, reduces fears and frustrations.

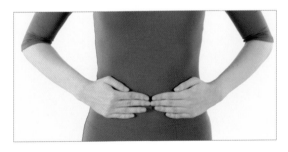

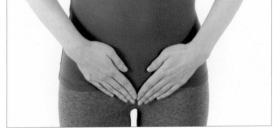

Position Three

Place your hands on either side of your navel, fingers touching. This position regulates sugar and fat metabolism (pancreas) and digestion, helps ease powerful emotions such as fears, depressions, and frustrations. It also helps to increase self-confidence.

Position Four

Place your hands over the pubic bone, in the shape of a "V". For women, the fingertips should touch. This position treats the large intestine, bladder, urethra, and sexual organs, eases menstrual disorders in woman, provides grounding, and helps existential fear.

TREATING YOUR BACK

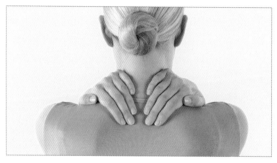

Position One

Place your hands on your upper shoulders, on either side of the spine. This position is helpful for shoulder tension, back and neck problems. It also promotes relaxation, releases blocked emotions, and helps problems with responsibility.

Position Two

Place one hand in the middle of your chest and the other at the same height on your back, palm facing outward. If you can't reach your shoulder blades, place your hands on your chest, one above the other. This balances the thymus gland, harmonizes the heart, stimulates the immune system and helps worries and depression.

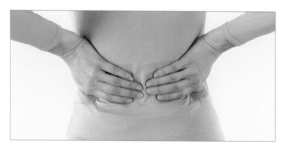

Position Three

Place your hands around your waist at kidney height, fingers pointing toward the spine. Strengthens kidneys, adrenal glands and nerves, promotes detoxification, relaxes stress, eases back pains, reinforces self-esteem and confidence.

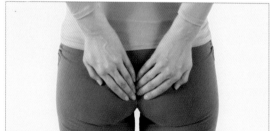

Position Four

Place your hands so that your fingers touch your coccyx, your hands opening into a "V". This position treats sexual organs, digestion, the sciatic nerve, promotes creativity and confidence, and provides grounding.

TREATING
OTHERS

It is best to give a full treatment and work through the basic positions. Remain in one hand position for between three and five minutes. In time, you will be able to sense exactly when a part of the body has received enough Reiki. Treat problem areas separately, for about ten or twenty minutes. At these points, you may experience heat or cold. Here, let your hands lie until you sense that the energy flow has normalized. If the energy is being well absorbed, you may feel tingling or throbbing in your hands.

Lay your hands gently and lightly on the receiver's body, keeping fingers together. Tell the receiver about possible self-healing reactions, which usually subside quickly. Give Reiki in emergencies and for shock and treat over the top of plaster casts. For burns, hold your hands just above the affected area.

For a complete treatment, allow between an hour and an hour and a half. Chronic complaints require intensive treatment, for several hours and over a prolonged period. With elderly or sick people, start with half an hour and then increase the time gradually. When treating babies and children, ten to twenty minutes may be sufficient.

Ideally, start with four treatments on four consecutive days. This allows the body enough time to open itself on an energetic plane and it is able to free itself of its toxins more effectively.

As it does so, chronic disorders may again become acute. These self-healing reactions are a part of the healing process and mostly subside again between two and twenty-four hours later. Blocked feelings may also be released and emotional reactions do occur. It is good to allow these emotions to express themselves.

After the four treatment days, give further treatments once or twice a week over several weeks. After each treatment remind the receiver to drink plenty, to eliminate toxins.

BEFORE EACH TREATMENT

Both the giver and receiver take off watches and jewelry.

The receiver should remove shoes, belts, and loosen tight clothing.

Cleanse the room with the First Symbol and charge it with positive energy.

Relax and center yourself, before starting the treatment.

The receiver should keep their legs uncrossed.

Play relaxing, meditative music or treat in silence.

Have a blanket ready in case of cold.

As the giver, remind yourself before and afterwards that you are being used as a channel for healing energy.

At the beginning and end smooth the aura three times from head to foot. At the end draw an energy line from the coccyx up over the head.

Wash your hands in cold running water afterwards to clear out energies.

Allow the receiver to rest for a while after the treatment has ended.

Aura smoothing

At the beginning of the treatment, stroke the receiver's aura in a smooth, curving form, starting at the head and working down to the feet. This has a relaxing effect on the receiver and prepares him or her for treatment.

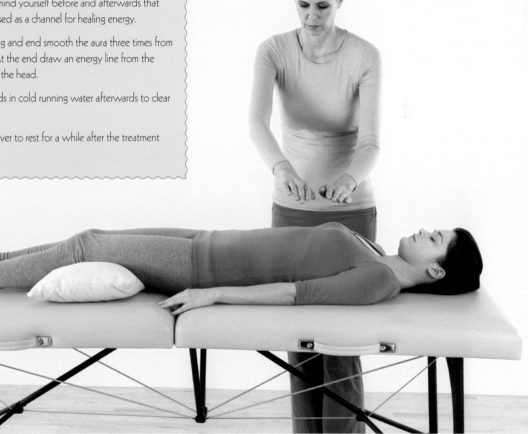

THE HEAD

It is usual to start a Reiki treatment by treating the head. The head positions have a strong effect, relaxing and balancing the whole body. Use a tissue for Head Position One, if your receiver wishes. Place it over the forehead and spread it out up to the tip of the nose.

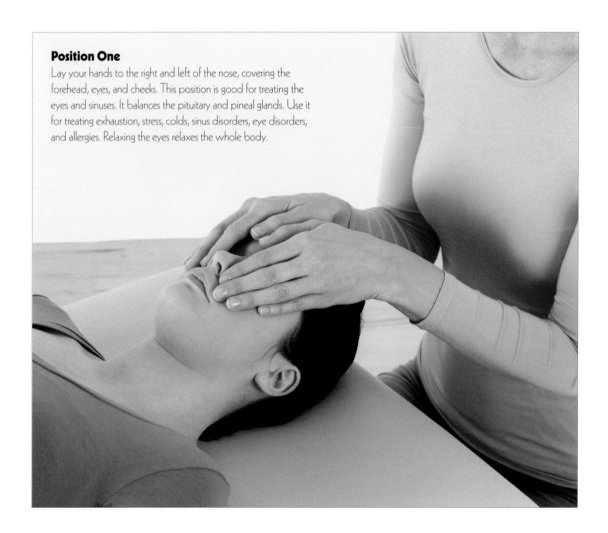

Position One
Lay your hands to the right and left of the nose, covering the forehead, eyes, and cheeks. This position is good for treating the eyes and sinuses. It balances the pituitary and pineal glands. Use it for treating exhaustion, stress, colds, sinus disorders, eye disorders, and allergies. Relaxing the eyes relaxes the whole body.

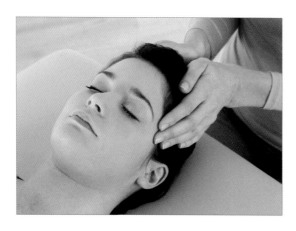

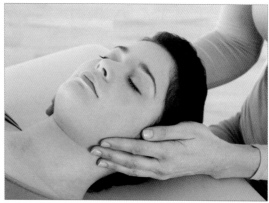

Position Two

Lay your hands on the temples, with the fingertips touching the cheekbones, the palms following the shape of the head. This position is good for treating the eye muscles and nerves. It balances the right and left sides of the brain, and the body. It helps ease stress, excessive mental activity and calms the mind, helps learning and concentration difficulties, alleviates colds, and headaches.

Position Three

Lay your hands over the ears. This position is good for treating the organs of balance and the pharynx. Use this to treat disturbances to the sense of balance, disorders of the outer and inner ear, noises or hissing in the ears, poor hearing, disorders of the nose and throat, and colds and flu.

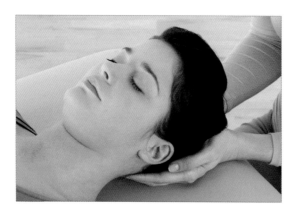

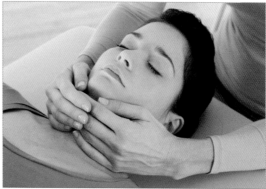

Position Four

Hold the back of the head with the fingertips over the medulla oblongata. This position is good for treating the back of the head, eyes, and nose and it helps to calm and clarify thinking. Use it for calming powerful emotions such as fear, shock, tension, headaches, eye disorders, colds, asthma, hayfever, and digestive disorders.

Position Five

Lay your hands at the sides and above the front part of the throat. Do not touch the throat directly. This treats the thyroid and parathyroid glands, larynx, vocal cords, and lymph nodes. Use it for metabolic disorders, weight problems, heart palpitations and fibrillation, high or low blood pressure, sore throat, inflammation of the tonsils, flu, hoarseness, aggression. Promotes self-expression.

FRONT OF BODY

By treating the front of the body, we deepen the whole healing process. Emotional reactions are quite possible, though they are not inevitable. As we apply Reiki here we balance the organs and stimulate the energy centres (chakras) on the front of the body.

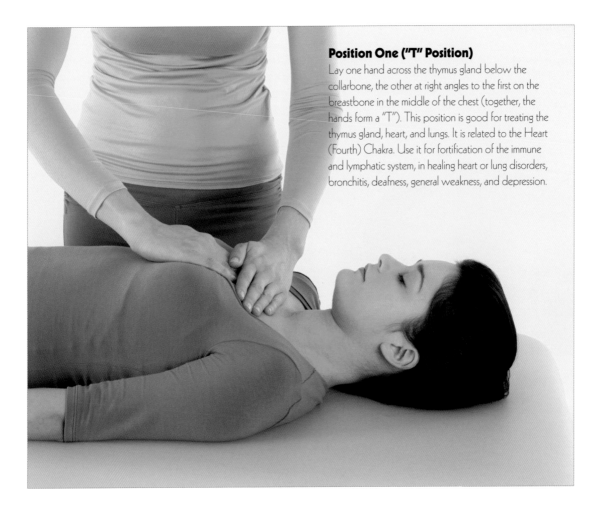

Position One ("T" Position)

Lay one hand across the thymus gland below the collarbone, the other at right angles to the first on the breastbone in the middle of the chest (together, the hands form a "T"). This position is good for treating the thymus gland, heart, and lungs. It is related to the Heart (Fourth) Chakra. Use it for fortification of the immune and lymphatic system, in healing heart or lung disorders, bronchitis, deafness, general weakness, and depression.

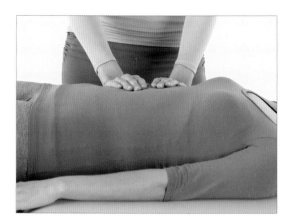

Position Two

Lay one hand on the lower ribs on the right side, below the chest; the other directly below it at waist level. This position is good for treating the liver and gallbladder, pancreas, duodenum, and parts of the stomach and large intestine. Use it for liver and gallbladder disorders, such as hepatitis, gall stones, digestive disorders, metabolic disorders, and detoxification problems. It also balances emotions such as anger and depression.

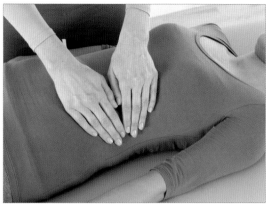

Position Three

Lay one hand on the lower ribs on the left side, below the chest, the other directly below it at waist level. This position is good for treating the spleen, parts of the pancreas, large intestine, small intestine, and stomach. Use it for disorders of the pancreas or spleen, diabetes, flu, infections, digestive disorders, anemia, and leukemia. In people with AIDS and cancer it helps to stabilize the immune system.

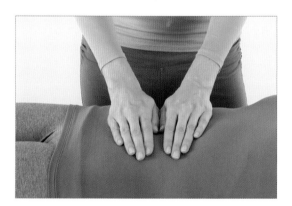

Position Four

Lay one hand above, and the other below, the navel. This position is good for treating the solar plexus, stomach, digestive organs, lymphatic system, and intestines. It is related to the Sacral (Second) and Solar Plexus (Third) Chakras. Use it for stomach and intestinal disorders, nausea, indigestion, bloated feelings, metabolic disorders, and powerful emotions such as depression, fears and shock. Good for restoring energy and vitality.

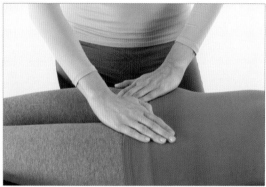

Position Five ("V" Position)

For men, place your hands in the groin area, without touching the sex organ. For women, lay both hands over the pubic bone. This position is good for treating the abdominal organs, intestines, bladder, and urethra. It is related to the Root (First) Chakra. Use it for urogenital, menstrual and menopausal disorders, appendix and digestive disorders, cramps, back pains, ovarian tumors, uterus, bladder, and prostate gland problems.

BACK OF BODY

Treating the back allows further letting go of tensions, thoughts, and feelings. By lying on the front of the body, the receiver feels more protected and so healing and relaxation can happen at deeper levels.

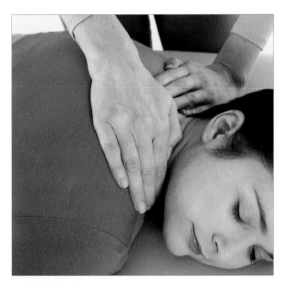

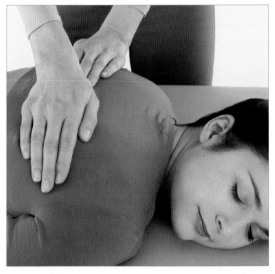

Position One

Lay both hands on the shoulders, one hand to the left and the other to the right of the spine. This position is good for treating the nape of the neck and the shoulder muscles. Use it for easing tension in the shoulders and the nape of the neck, neck problems, stress, blocked emotions, and problems with responsibility.

Position Two

Lay your hands on the shoulder blades. This position is good for treating shoulders, heart, lungs, and upper back. Use it for lung and heart disorders, coughs, bronchitis, back and shoulder complaints, powerful emotional upsets, and depression. Promotes capacity for love, confidence, and enjoyment.

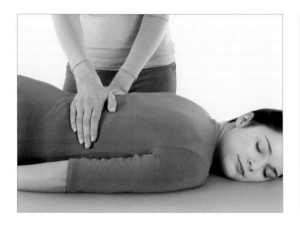

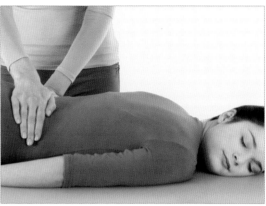

Position Three

Lay your hands on the lower ribs above the kidneys. This position helps in the treatment of the adrenal glands, kidneys, and nervous system. Use it for kidney disorders, allergies, detoxification, hayfever, shock from emergencies and accidents, fears, stress, and back pains. By releasing the middle back we let go of the past, of stress and pain.

Position Four

If the receiver has a long back, lay your hands on the lower part of the back (at hip level). This position helps with sciatica and lower back pain, strengthens the lymph and nerves, supports creativity and sexuality, and eases hip problems.

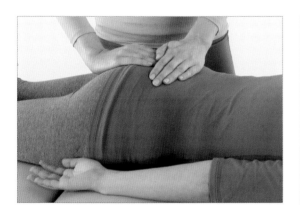

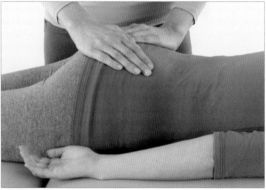

Position Five (A) or "T" Position

Lay one hand across the sacrum, the other at right angles to the first, over the coccyx to form a "T". This position is good for treating the intestines, the urogenital system, and the sciatic nerve. It is related to the Root (First) Chakra. It helps existential fears. Use it for hemorrhoids, digestive complaints, intestinal inflammations, bladder disorders, prostate gland problems, vaginal disorders, and sciatic pain.

Position Five (B) or "V" Position

Lay the fingertips of one hand directly on the coccyx (sometimes you will have to feel around a bit to find this bone), and lay the other hand next to the first to form a "V". The treatment is the same as for Back Position Five (A) or "T" Position. With the fingertips directly on the coccyx the energy can more easily travel along the spine (upward); it energizes and harmonizes the nervous system, promoting confidence.

THE LEGS

The legs and feet carry the whole weight of the body. Problems with the legs, knees, and feet can indicate a hesitation and fear of moving forward in life. We also store emotions in the upper and lower leg areas. By applying Reiki we release this energy and can bring awareness to take the right steps in the right direction.

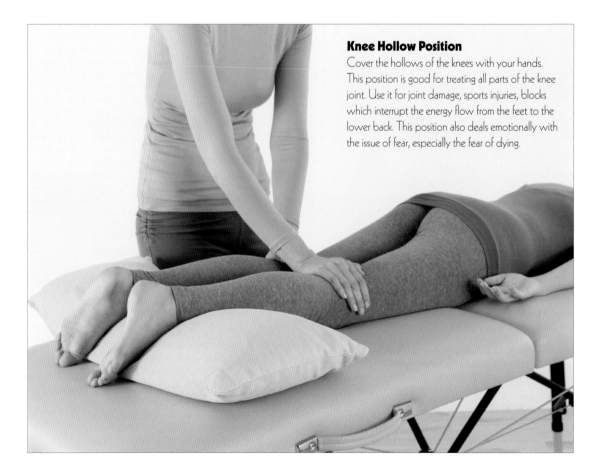

Knee Hollow Position
Cover the hollows of the knees with your hands. This position is good for treating all parts of the knee joint. Use it for joint damage, sports injuries, blocks which interrupt the energy flow from the feet to the lower back. This position also deals emotionally with the issue of fear, especially the fear of dying.

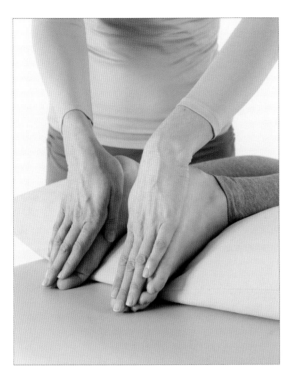

Sole Position (A)

Lay your hands on the soles of the feet, ideally with your fingertips covering the toes. The Sole Positions are good for treating the foot reflex zones for all organs which are located over the whole sole of the foot. Use these positions for fortification of the Root (First) Chakra and grounding of all chakras and regions of the body.

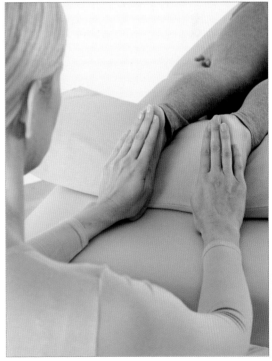

Sole Position (B)

Rest the balls of your hands on the toes and point your fingertips toward the heels. This position has the same effect as Sole Position (A). The receiver will sense a strengthened energy flow from feet to head, and the body is experienced as a whole.

"I have found that Reiki has improved me in every facet of my life. On the health side the eczema on my legs has cleared."
JUDY

ADDITIONAL
POSITIONS

These positions are useful to try out whenever you experience a specific problem that you want to concentrate on exclusively. This can include, for example, sciatic pain, neck problems, or the inability to release pent-up emotions and tensions that are being held in the body.

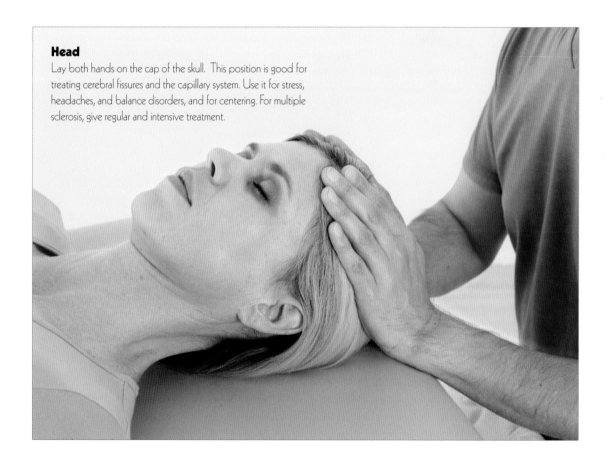

Head

Lay both hands on the cap of the skull. This position is good for treating cerebral fissures and the capillary system. Use it for stress, headaches, and balance disorders, and for centering. For multiple sclerosis, give regular and intensive treatment.

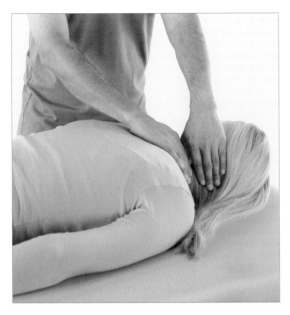

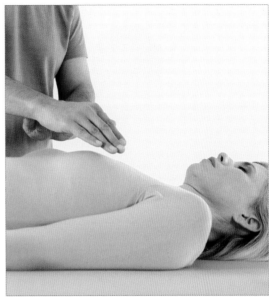

Neck Vertebrae

Lay one hand on the nape of the neck and the other on the top neck vertebra. Use this position for whiplash injury, pain in the bones, heart, spine, nerve, and neck problems.

Breast/Chest

Lay the hands over both sides of the chest. This position helps to harmonize the male and female sides.

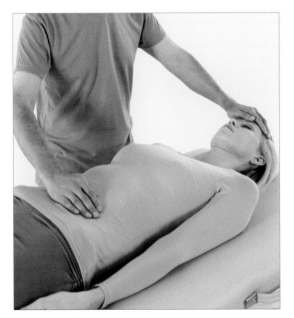

Head and Belly

Lay one hand on the forehead and the other on the belly (just below the navel). This position has a calming and centering effect, it promotes spiritual equilibrium, and relaxes those suffering from stress and shock.

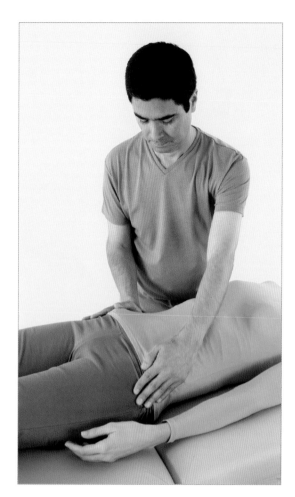

Hip Joints

Lay your hands on the left and right hips. This position is good for treating hip joints, varicose veins, leg pain, and the gall point of the meridian system in the body.

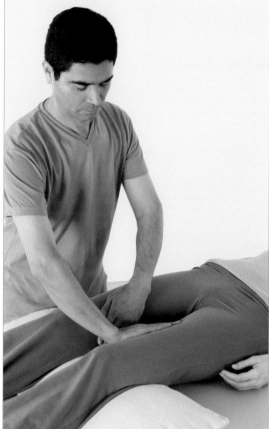

Thighs

Lay one hand flat on the inside of each thigh (fingertips pointing in opposite directions). This position is effective for treating the intestines. Emotions and tensions are released. This is a let-go position for deep-seated fears.

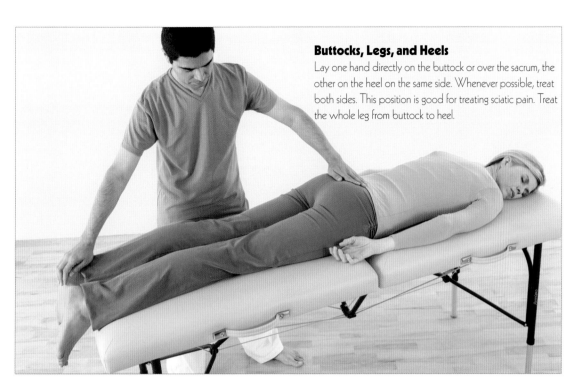

Buttocks, Legs, and Heels

Lay one hand directly on the buttock or over the sacrum, the other on the heel on the same side. Whenever possible, treat both sides. This position is good for treating sciatic pain. Treat the whole leg from buttock to heel.

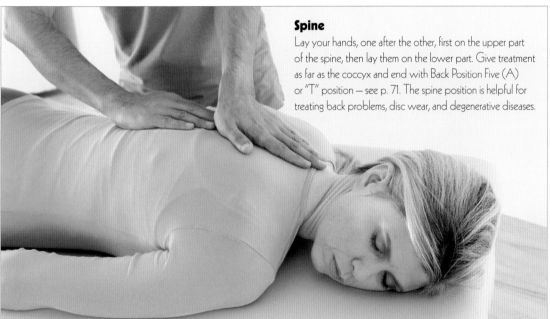

Spine

Lay your hands, one after the other, first on the upper part of the spine, then lay them on the lower part. Give treatment as far as the coccyx and end with Back Position Five (A) or "T" position — see p. 71. The spine position is helpful for treating back problems, disc wear, and degenerative diseases.

REIKI SHORT
TREATMENT

This treatment is useful for stressful situations and headaches, for balancing the chakras, if there is no time for a full treatment, or if the receiver is tense and needs an energetic refresher. The receiver sits comfortably, legs uncrossed, hands resting on thighs. At the beginning and end, stroke the aura from head to foot (see p. 65). This calms and refreshes, especially if you take the last stroke from the sacral region up over the head. As a first-aid measure for shock, use Positions Ten and Eleven.

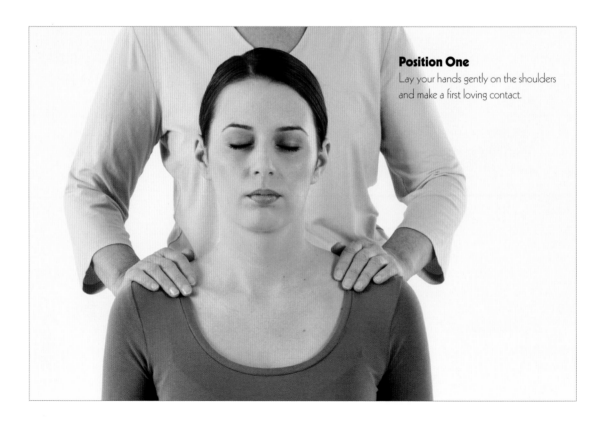

Position One
Lay your hands gently on the shoulders and make a first loving contact.

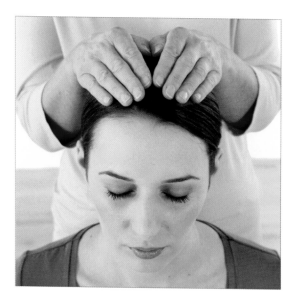

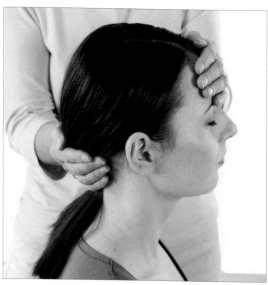

Position Two

Lay your hands on the cap of the skull, leaving the Crown (Seventh) Chakra free.

Position Three

Lay one hand on the medulla oblongata (transition from the back of the head to the spine), the other on the forehead.

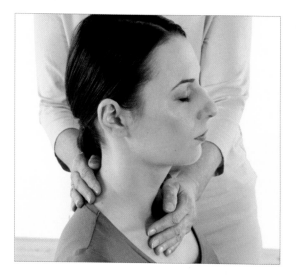

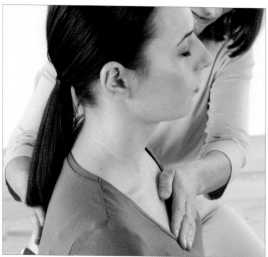

Position Four

Lay one hand on the seventh neck vertebra (projecting vertebra), the other on the hollow below the Adam's apple.

Position Five

Lay one hand on the Heart (Fourth) Chakra at the center of the chest (breast bone/heart center), the other at the same height on the back between the shoulder blades.

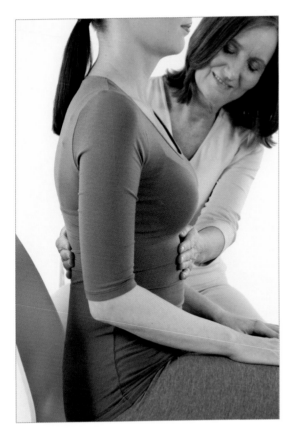

Position Six
Lay one hand on the stomach covering the Solar Plexus (Third) Chakra, the other at the same height on the back.

Position Seven
Lay one hand below the navel, the other at the same height on the back (the sacral region). You can end with this position or, if you still have a few minutes, Positions Eight and Nine are good for treating the knees and feet.

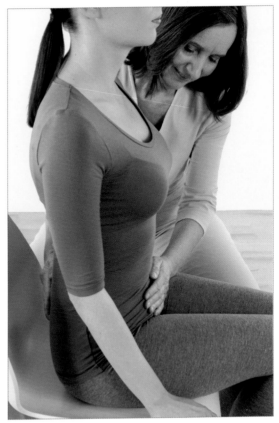

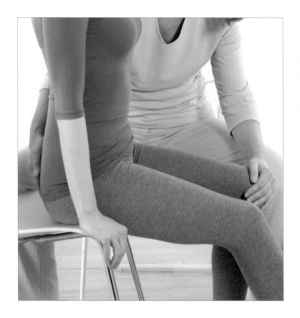

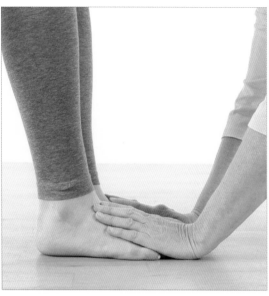

Position Eight

Lay one hand on the sacrum at the Root (First) Chakra, with your fingertips pointing downward and the other on one knee. Then change sides and treat the other knee.

Position Nine

Lay your hands on the feet with the fingertips covering the tops of the feet and the heels of your hands resting on the floor.

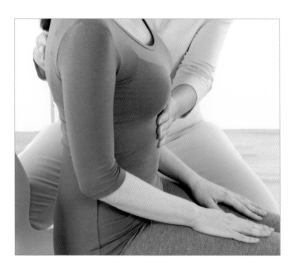

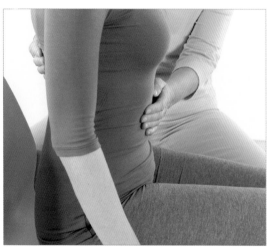

Position Ten

Lay one hand on the upper back between the shoulder blades (at heart height), the other at the front on the solar plexus.

Position Eleven

Lay one hand on the middle of the back or on the waist (over the kidneys and adrenal glands), the other at the front on the stomach.

MENTAL
HEALING

In Mental Healing, the giver makes contact, using the Reiki Symbols (see pp. 38–40), with the hidden regions of consciousness. The Second Symbol connects you directly with the receiver's superconscious, known as the Higher Self, and subconscious through which you learn more about programing, conditioning, and the causes of problems and illnesses. Mental Healing can help you to transform misdirected energies so that the receiver can experience optimism, love, and happiness.

During this kind of healing, knowledge is passed from the subconscious to the waking consciousness in different forms. Messages of sudden insight appear and the causes of problems are recognized. For example, reading a passage in a book may unexpectedly resonate with your problem: you receive the message you need to hear. Fears, addictions, and other mental or spiritual disturbances can be influenced positively. This is particularly helpful in discovering the spiritual and mental causes of physical illnesses. Mental Healing offers an opportunity to gain more awareness of past conditioning and programing. This is a first step toward healing. The more aware you become of what you think of yourself and what state your self-esteem is in, the more you become aware of your programing and fixed belief pattern. Mental Healing encourages you to seek more clarity in your life. For example,

what do you want to invite and integrate into your life? Mental healing demands great responsibility from the giver since it brings you into direct contact with the receiver's subconscious and superconscious. All messages you send on the mental level are registered by the receiver's subconscious. Your mind must be clear, calm, and empty. To clear out your mind try the Gibberish Meditation (see facing page). Carry out Mental Healing only if you have the receiver's consent and use it for his or her own benefit alone.

For a Mental Healing session the receiver sits on a chair. The sequence takes about fifteen minutes and can be incorporated into a normal Reiki treatment. You can also give yourself Mental Healing either in the morning or evening before bed. By treating yourself with Mental Healing you deepen your connection with your own subconscious and Higher Self.

"During mental healing I felt very open. Suddenly, as if a light bulb had gone on inside me, I understood the things which had previously been unclear."

HENRY

AFFIRMATIONS

In Mental Healing you can work with affirmations, decided on together. These describe a positive state that you wish for yourself. You visualize this positive state. This can include parts of the body, feelings, and states of mind. The following affirmations, or ones like it, can be very powerful:

1. "I (say your name) love myself, simply because I am as I am." This opens up your heart and the whole burden of fighting and rejecting yourself may dissolve in a gentle, tearful manner. Speaking this affirmation brings you back closer to yourself again. In this state you can love and accept yourself. This affirmation embraces all three areas: mind, body, and spirit.

2. If you are working on one area only, use the following: "I (name) now love and accept my body."

3. If you are working on the emotions, use the following: "I (name) open up my heart and now accept all my feelings."

4. If you are working in the mental area, use the following: "My meditation is getting deeper every day."

GIBBERISH MEDITATION

The mind thinks in words, so babbling helps you to get rid of thoughts. Let your body express itself, too, by shaking your hands and head. Do this alone or in a group. This is a good way to relax before Mental Healing.

1. Close your eyes and start to "babble": blurt out noises without thinking, as if you were speaking a foreign language which you do not understand.

2. Lose yourself in babble for 15 minutes. Allow yourself to express anything that wants to come out. Let your body be expressive also.

3. Afterward lie on your front for 15 minutes and feel yourself melting into the floor every time you breathe out.

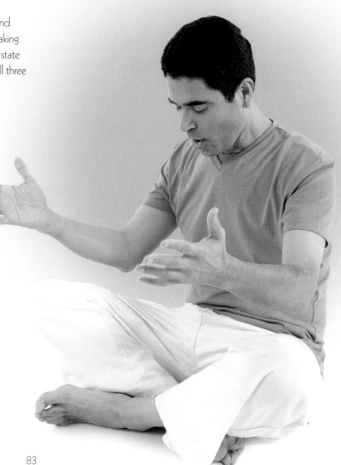

DISTANT
HEALING

This form of healing is an essential part of the Second Degree. It lets you send mental messages and healing forces over a distance. This is similar to the phenomenon of thought transference. How often have you thought about someone and then received a letter or phone call from him or her that very day? An incident like this may seem like mere coincidence, but it is proof that thoughts are transmitted and received on the mental level (telepathy).

Rather like radio and television technology, we use the phenomenon of "wireless" transmission in Distant Healing. We know that the vibrations of radio and television signals, invisible to the human eye, are transmitted through space. With the help of the Third Symbol (see p.40), you can use a similar type of energy transference to make mental contact with people who are not physically present.

You apply the method of Distant Healing with an appropriate visualization technique (see also pp. 54–5) and transmit the healing energy to the receiver as if over a "bridge of light". In this way, you can transmit vital energy over long distances. The healing power may be greatly amplified during Distant Healing because mental forces are very strong. However, receivers usually experience contact treatment more distinctly even though the kind of energy in both cases

is essentially the same (though with different degrees of intensity). As the giver, you sense very distinctly the different flows of energy moving into the different parts of the receiver's body. You may also gain a clear idea of what is wrong with the receiver and how he or she is absorbing the treatment. It is a good idea to make a few notes after a Distant Healing treatment of things that you may want to tell the receiver about in a subsequent telephone call, e-mail or letter.

Ideally, you and the receiver should agree the treatment time for a Distant Healing in advance and the receiver should sit or lie down, since it is better for him or her not to be doing anything. If you don't know your receiver personally, use a photograph of him or her to help visualize where you will be focusing your attention. Usually a Distant Healing session takes between fifteen and thirty minutes.

You can use Distant Healing whenever, for reasons of time or distance, you are unable to meet the receiver. For example, if the receiver has to have an operation, you can treat them before and after (but not during) the operation (see also p. 54). You should never carry out a treatment against someone's will.

If you have not been able to arrange a specific time, ask the person at the start of your contact with them they want to receive distant healing from you. This also applies in the case of a previously agreed arrangement between friends. Always ask for permission and do not intrude. It is also important to be aware of so-called "helper trips" (when it makes you feel good to help others, so that your motives are suspect). Reiki is a non-intrusive healing method. If people do not want to receive it, then you should respect their wishes. In general, the best advice is to wait until you are asked before you send Reiki.

You can send yourself Distant Healing or find things out for yourself at any time. Using the techniques of Distant Healing, you can send healing and light into specific problem areas and difficult or unresolved situations. Using the Second and Third Symbols (see p. 40) you can combine Mental and Distant Healing methods. You can also work on and heal themes going back into the more distant past, such as traumatic events in childhood (see also p. 106).

With Distant Healing, you can give Reiki to other people, to animals (see pp. 94–5), and to plants (see p. 92). Get together with some Reiki friends and allow thoughts of peace and healing energies to flow to the whole planet. Using Reiki together in a group creates a more powerful energy field (see pp. 116–17). The exact procedure for Distant Healing is taught in the course of the Second Degree seminar.

Healing the planet

In times of general unrest, during disasters and wars, you can send Reiki to the whole Earth, or concentrate on a specific region.

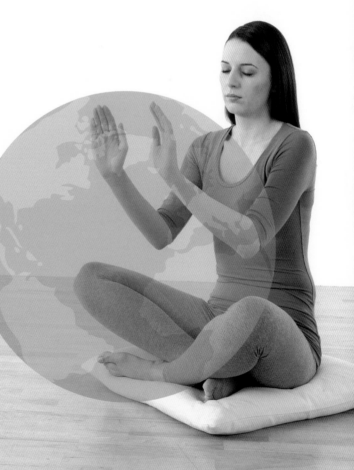

HARMONIZING
CHAKRAS

The balancing of the energy centers (chakras) with Reiki is very effective. As the basic Reiki positions follow the seven main chakras, which are numbered One to Seven, you can easily integrate the harmonization of the chakras into a single Reiki treatment. You can also treat the energy centers separately. This takes about fifteen to twenty minutes.

Each chakra reflects an aspect of personal growth. If we have a block in the energy flow of our chakras, this may lead to an imbalance and to a mental-spiritual or physical disorder. The positions of the individual chakras are shown on the chart (see pp. 88–9), which describes the corresponding organs and characteristics of the chakras. With the help of Reiki you can harmonize, or balance out, an excess or shortage of energy in your chakras.

As a rule there is often too much energy in the head and too little in the lower body. The Crown (Seventh) Chakra does not need any additional energy, so you do not touch it in the course of harmonizing the chakras.

If you lay one hand on the Root (First) Chakra and the other on the forehead, or Third Eye (Sixth), you can correct this imbalance easily. To do this, allow the hands to rest on these two points until you can feel the same energy in both chakras. You may feel

a temperature difference at the two points, ranging from warm to cold, so wait until you feel both hands becoming equally warm. Then lay one hand on the Throat (Fifth) Chakra and the other on the Sacral (Second) Chakra (see illustration). Here, too, you leave both hands in place until you sense the same amount of energy is flowing in both of them.

Then lay one hand on the Heart (Fourth) Chakra in the middle of the chest, and the other on the Solar Plexus (Third) Chakra. Let your hands rest until you sense equal energy flowing in both of them.

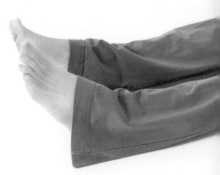

You can also bring the chakras back into equilibrium by laying one hand on the Root (First) Chakra and balancing all the other chakras with it, one after the other. The same applies for the Third Eye (Sixth) Chakra. Leave one hand resting on the forehead and lay the other on all the chakras, one after the other. This is a good balancing treatment when you have too much energy in your head and would like to move some of it down to the lower chakras. You can reinforce the harmonization of the chakras by using the corresponding Symbol (see pp. 38–40). (See also pp. 30–1.)

"I have often felt scared to open some of my Pandora's boxes, but now I feel excited about working through these things."
ELAINE

A harmonization example
This photograph shows the hand positions for harmonizing the Throat (Fifth) and Sacral (Second) Chakras.

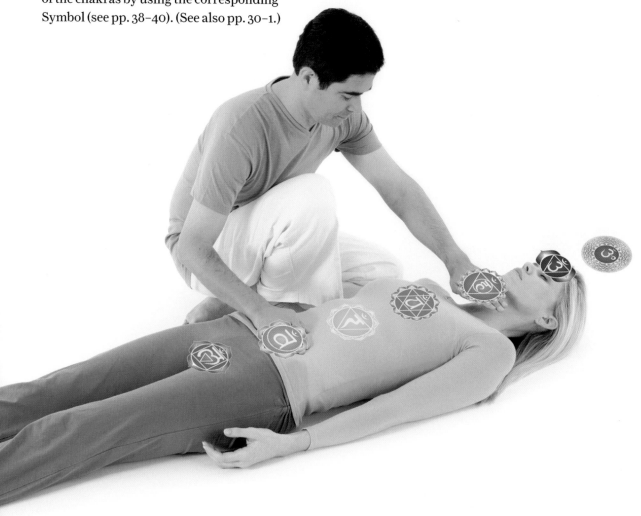

THE CHAKRAS: CORRESPONDING ORGANS

Chakra	Name	Organs
	CROWN (7th) CHAKRA	Upper brain, right eye, pineal gland
	THIRD EYE (6th) CHAKRA	Lower brain, left eye, nose, spine, ears, pituitary gland
	THROAT (5th) CHAKRA	Throat, thyroid gland, upper lungs and arms, digestive tract
	HEART (4th) CHAKRA	Heart, lungs, circulation, thymus gland
	SOLAR PLEXUS (3rd) CHAKRA	Stomach, liver, gallbladder, pancreas, solar plexus
	SACRAL (2nd) CHAKRA	Reproductive organs, urogenital system, kidneys, gonads, legs
	ROOT (1st) CHAKRA	Adrenal glands, bladder, genitals, spine

CORRESPONDING THEMES

Themes   **Chakra**

Consciousness of oneness, spiritual awareness, extended
consciousness, wisdom, intuition, connection to the Higher Self, to the
inner guidance, and to all-embracing love

Clairvoyance, telepathy, seat of the will, thought control, inner vision
and understanding, inspiration, spiritual awakening

Self-expression, communication, creativity, sense of responsibility

Center of the emotions, love for self and others, peace, sympathy,
forgiveness, trust, spiritual development, compassion

Power, dominance, strength, fear

Vitality, enjoyment of life, self-esteem, refinement of feelings,
relationships, desire

Will to live, life force, survival, fertility, procreation

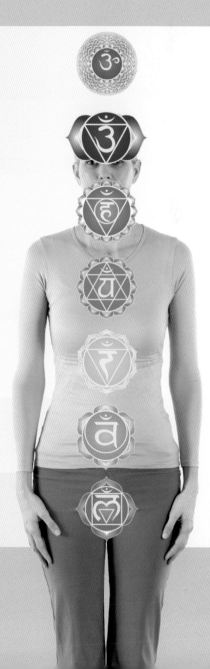

GROUNDING

To have "good grounding" means that you are connected to the Earth; you have "both feet on the ground". You are centered inside yourself and are well "rooted", or connected with the Root (First) Chakra. This exercise is good to try when you want to ground yourself and take up more Earth energy. Whenever you are living "in your head" too much (thinking too hard rather than "living in the present moment"), have too many thoughts, fears, and worries, you lack contact with yourself and connection with "Mother Earth". It is also good to do this exercise before Reiki healing treatments in order to strengthen your presence and your rootedness.

ENERGIZING YOUR CHAKRAS

1. Stand relaxed and comfortable, with your feet shoulder width apart. Close your eyes.

2. Breathe in deeply and, when you breathe out, let your shoulders hang loose and relaxed. Repeat this two or three times, each time releasing tensions in your body when you breathe out.

3. Now concentrate on your feet. Imagine you are taking up energy from the Earth. While you breathe in, allow Earth energy to flow into the left foot. You can also imagine drawing the energy up from the center of the Earth. This energy flows up your left leg and through the Root (First) Chakra (this lies low in the pelvis and opens to the Earth below).

4. While you are breathing out imagine the Earth energy flowing down your right leg and through your right foot back into the Earth. Imagine the energy flowing back to the center of the Earth. After five to ten minutes, end the exercise here, or carry on.

5. If you carry on, let Earth energy flow into you through the left foot and the left leg as you breathe in. Then let it flow through the Sacral (Second) Chakra and back down the right leg and right foot into the Earth, while you breathe out. Treat all seven chakras, from the Root (First) up to the Crown (Seventh). Allow the Earth energy to flow through each chakra for about two minutes.

"I use Reiki to balance my own energies and nourish myself. It helps me on my spiritual journey."
KARIN

"*I am completely sold on Reiki and it is the only satisfactory way of relaxing that I have, so far, experienced.*"
BRIAN

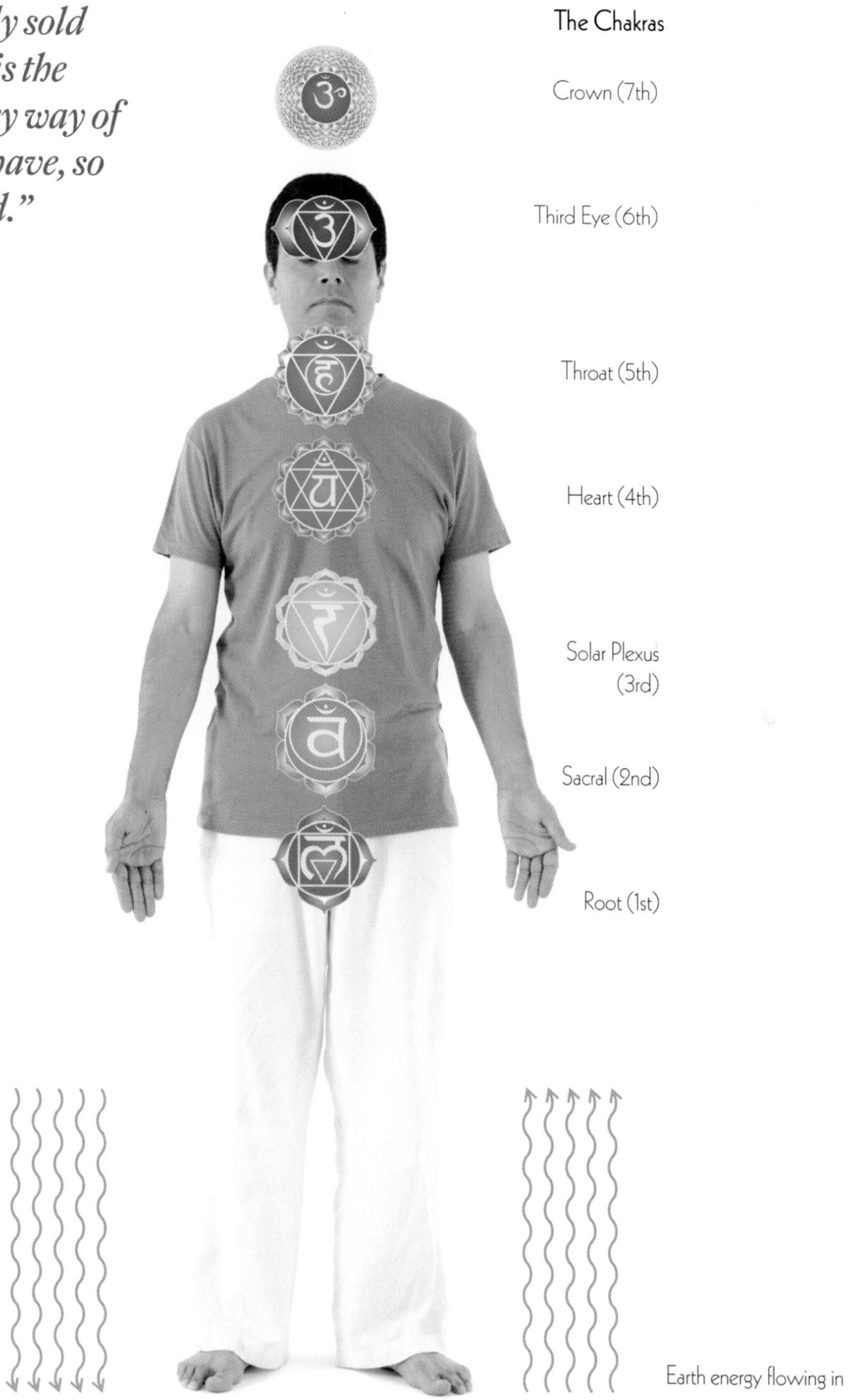

The Chakras

Crown (7th)

Third Eye (6th)

Throat (5th)

Heart (4th)

Solar Plexus (3rd)

Sacral (2nd)

Root (1st)

Earth energy flowing out

Earth energy flowing in

6. REIKI IN DAILY LIFE

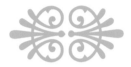

The Universal Life Energy, or Reiki, is a powerful natural energy which flows through all of us. It is the basic energy which created us all and flows constantly through all living beings – humans, animals, and plants – nourishing and sustaining them. This energy is available to all and is drawn on and used up in our daily activities. By applying Reiki, we can replenish this energy and bring about bodily, emotional, and mental equilibrium.

Reiki can be used effectively on everything which lives. The consciousness of animals and plants is not the same as human consciousness, but we all share natural growth cycles, health, sickness, and death. Plants and animals also suffer, just as we do, from the effects of environmental pollution and are exposed to accidents and stressful situations. Reiki can help ease the effects of all of these.

Reiki for Plants

Just as the Universal Life Energy manifests itself in humans and animals, it is also manifested in plants, which respond very positively to Reiki treatment. This is revealed in health, strong growth, good blossom, and long life. You can give potted plants Reiki in the root area by putting your hands around the whole flower pot. You can also give Reiki directly to the roots or to an injured stem. If you want to repot a plant, treat the roots before you replant it. In the case of seeds, hold them in your hand for a few minutes before sowing them. You can also continue to give Reiki when the seeds have already been sown. In the case of seedlings, treat the roots for a few minutes. For cut flowers, hold the stems and, later, place your hands around the whole vase.

If you wish, try giving Reiki to trees. Put your arms right around the tree if you can. Otherwise lay your hands on the trunk or on the earth surrounding the trunk. After such a treatment, you may feel as though you are "charged up", harmonious, and strengthened. It is better to treat sick forests with Distant Healing (see pp. 84–5). You can treat your whole garden in the same way. Regular treatment of your vegetable or fruit garden will reward you with a wealth of healthy, sturdy plants and plenty of good quality fruit.

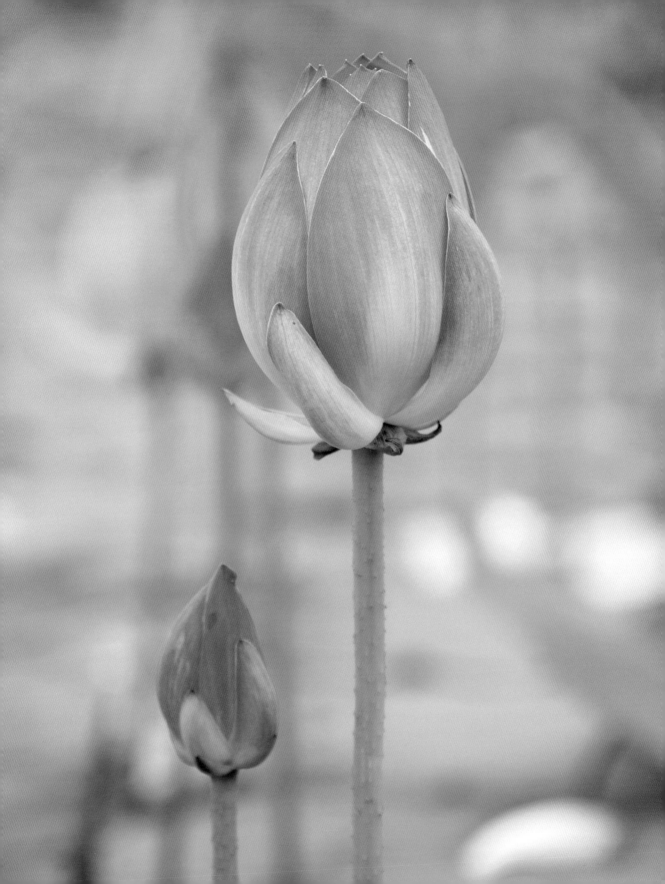

"Birds in shock respond very well to the healing warmth of Reiki. They will close their eyes for a few minutes before they suddenly fly away."

ALISON

Reiki for Animals

Animals seem to like receiving Reiki and sense immediately that something special is being given to them by human hands. It is very unusual to come across animals who do not accept Reiki energy; often they become calm and relaxed in the course of a treatment and this is something to be respected by humans. Usually, animals show you with their body position where to place your hands. If you want to treat a certain internal organ, you can assume, in the case of mammals, that its position is roughly the same as in humans. Most pets (such as cats and dogs) and domestic animals have a similar anatomical structure to ours. In every treatment pay attention to areas of the body which draw a greater amount of energy. Spend more time here than at other neutral positions, just as you would if you were treating a person. It is always a good idea to treat an animal's endocrine glands (see p. 30).

Cats and dogs and other animals tend to remain lying down for as long as they need Reiki and they will generally stand up or jump away when they have had enough. Twenty or thirty minutes' treatment is usually sufficient.

For animals who have undergone an operation, Reiki can be very beneficial if you give it directly afterwards. Subsequent daily treatments can then speed up recovery considerably. Before operations and before anesthesia, Reiki is highly recommended for both large and small animals. They willingly accept the calming effect of Reiki hands. Their breathing slows down and their heartbeat becomes regular. Reiki also helps them to recover far more quickly from the anesthetic.

It may be possible to calm a restless, excited animal by stroking it and talking to it gently, but if not, treat it with Distant Healing (see pp. 84–5). This also applies to zoo animals or those that are too dangerous to touch. If you treat larger domesticated animals, such as cows or horses, you can lay your hands directly on the place where the problem is.

In general animals like being touched on the head – behind the ears, under the chin, and in the middle of the forehead above the eyes. You can also treat the belly, chest, back, and organs as necessary. For fish and birds, lay your hands around the whole aquarium or birdcage. You can hold small birds in one hand and lay the other hand around them. Animals in emergency situations and disasters, and species threatened with extinction can most effectively be treated with Distant Healing.

Because of close cohabitation with humans, pets increasingly tend to suffer from human-style illnesses such as colds, allergies, and tumors. Just as we suffer from stress, pets can suffer similarly, experiencing negative effects on the immune system. Today, there are more and more veterinary surgeons keen to try alternative and complementary healing methods such as homeopathy, Bach Flower

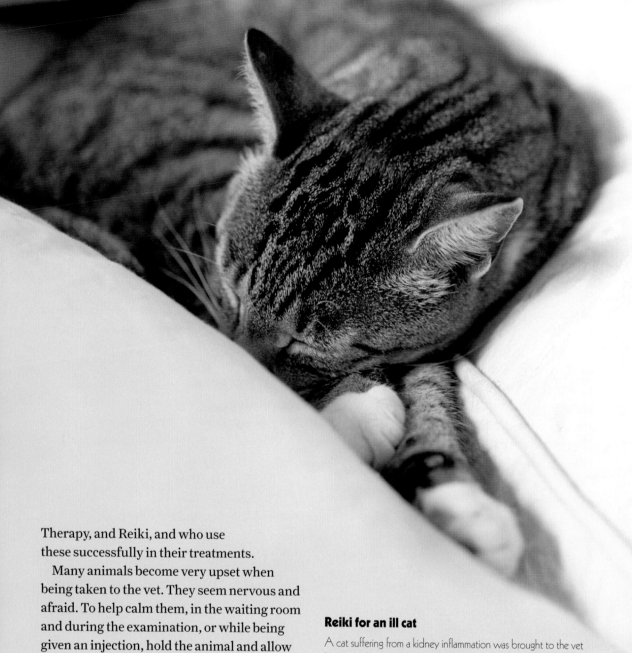

Therapy, and Reiki, and who use
these successfully in their treatments.

Many animals become very upset when
being taken to the vet. They seem nervous and
afraid. To help calm them, in the waiting room
and during the examination, or while being
given an injection, hold the animal and allow
Reiki to flow into it. During the examination,
animals seem to be less anxious if they are
touched by Reiki hands. You can help to
soothe and harmonize their powerful
emotional reactions.

Reiki for an ill cat

A cat suffering from a kidney inflammation was brought to the vet
by its owner. It had become very thin and its major organs were
no longer functioning properly. Its owner wanted to have it put
to sleep. The assistant, trained in Reiki, immediately began to treat
the cat. It had hardly any life energy and could scarcely eat. But
after daily treatment with Reiki for a week, it was fit enough to
go home.

REIKI
FIRST AID

In emergency situations, the body automatically goes into a "fight or flight" reaction. The adrenal cortex increases production of the hormone adrenalin, which supports our reaction to stress. The adrenalin is transported in the blood to the body's cells, making the person wide awake and ready to react. However, the adrenal glands are soon exhausted and are then under tension and stress. You can help the adrenal glands in emergency situations by calming and balancing them with Reiki.

During the treatment, you can also lay one hand, in front, on the Solar Plexus (Third) Chakra and the other at the same height on the back in Position Six of the Short Treatment, (see p. 80). This reduces the effects of shock. For a calming effect, you can also lay one hand on the back of the head (medulla oblongata) and the other hand on the Third Eye (Sixth) Chakra. If the nature of the situation or the position of the accident victim makes it impossible to touch the parts of the body affected, you can also hold one or both of the person's hands.

In the case of an accident always phone for a doctor first of all and then use Reiki to calm the injured person while you are waiting. If the person is unconscious, do not attempt to move them because of possible spine or neck injury.

As the injured person is likely to be in shock, lay your hands on the front of the body on the Solar Plexus (Third) Chakra or on the back in the region of the kidneys and adrenal glands (see p. 30).

"When I first heard that Reiki could stop bleeding, I was a little sceptical, but an accident convinced me otherwise. A deep wound on my wrist landed me in hospital. I immediately laid my hand over it and found that the wound was hardly bleeding at all."

LESLEY

FEAR

Lay your hands on the Solar Plexus (Third) Chakra, adrenal glands, and the back of the head and carry out Mental Healing (see pp. 82–3).

INSECT BITES

Give Reiki directly on the bite for 20 or 30 minutes. If you can give Reiki immediately, you may be able to keep the swelling down.

BROKEN BONES

Before you give Reiki directly to the fracture point, this should first be set by a doctor. Then you can lay your hands gently on the plaster.

SPRAINS

Give Reiki to the injured area for 30 to 60 minutes, repeating several times according to the severity of the sprain.

BURNS

Give Reiki just above, not touching, the actual injury, for 20 or 30 minutes, possibly at intervals. The pain may initially worsen before beginning to subside. If you can give Reiki straight away, blisters are less likely.

HEART ATTACK

Call a doctor immediately. In the meantime, give Reiki to the upper and lower belly, but not directly to the heart.

WOUNDS

Give Reiki just above the wound. Later, after the dressing has been applied, give Reiki through the bandage.

SHOCK/ACCIDENT

Call a doctor immediately. In the meantime give Reiki to the Solar Plexus (Third) Chakra and the adrenal glands simultaneously, and later to the shoulders.

BRUISING

Give Reiki immediately, directly on the bruise, for 20 or 30 minutes.

"Since the Second Degree there has been a tremendous clearing of emotional and mental aspects of my life. Reiki is working through me."

BOB

REIKI FOR
EVERYDAY STRESS

Stress is generally thought to be the reaction of the body to the demands of daily life. If you cannot cope with these, you may react with physical, emotional, and mental stress symptoms. If you suffer stress over a prolonged period, the body loses vitality and resilience. You become susceptible to illnesses; you worry, become fearful, depressed or angry, exhausted, and irritable; you become confused, and are unable to think clearly, or make the right decisions. Spiritually, you may feel empty, find no enjoyment in life, and feel bored.

LAUGHTER MEDITATION

You can do this with your eyes open or closed.

1. When you wake up in the morning, stretch and arch your whole body like a cat, even before you open your eyes.

2. After a couple of minutes, start to laugh. Simply lift the corners of your mouth and laugh, even if you do not feel like it. Soon the forced laughter will stimulate the real thing and your laughter will become quite spontaneous. This will change your mood for the day.

If stress mounts up, this accumulation leads to continuing disturbances in the physical-spiritual area. Common symptoms of stress are difficulties in falling and staying asleep, headaches, unwarranted fears, feeling "wound up", chronic fatigue, concentration and learning difficulties, worrying, irritability, stomach pains, digestive problems, colds, outbursts of anger, and excessive eating, drinking, and smoking. These reactions can affect relationships at work and in private life.

In the case of sadness, anger, depression, fear, frustration, hate, guilt, self-pity, and loneliness, Reiki helps you attain and keep inner strength and clarity. You learn to accept feelings and to go through painful processes and come out strengthened.

Underlying Pain
Reiki helps you to experience your anger, fear, or feelings of guilt, and to make contact with underlying pain. In so doing, you open your heart, begin to love yourself, and let go of negative emotions. When you recognize and understand the causes of these emotions, you learn to transform them. Fear and anger become trust, love, and connectedness. Depression and guilt turn into enjoyment of life, vitality, and courage. You are able to search inside yourself and explore places where you might be holding on to negative feelings. That is where you lay your hands.

With Reiki, you can bring negative feelings into harmony with a higher energy vibration. Universal Life Energy lets you transform feelings with lower frequencies into positive feelings with higher frequency.

"I had a wonderful feeling of peace and tranquility and a feeling of empowerment and self-centeredness."
GILL

Suppressing Emotion
Most people suppress their negative feelings. They would prefer not to know about them. When you repress these dark emotions, you use up life force energy. Since you do not want to feel, you also cut yourself off from positive emotions. By using Reiki regularly, you can develop well-being and harmony on all levels. Your body is vital and healthy and you feel emotionally and mentally balanced. You learn to take over responsibility for your health and well-being.

The saying "laughter is the best medicine" has more than a grain of truth (see facing page). Laughing stimulates the thymus gland, strengthening the immune system. If you laugh often, you see things from a more positive viewpoint and do not take yourself so seriously. You no longer identify with your problems so strongly. Laughter rocks the heart, letting it release negative energies. It also vitalizes the body, simply because you breathe more deeply when you are laughing. It massages the heart and is the best medicine there is. Laughter is infectious!

Reiki for Emotional Problems
When you experience negative emotions within yourself or in others, try to lay your hands

directly on the place where you or the receiver feels the emotion. The head positions calm your thoughts and your moods. They bring you into contact with positive qualities such as trust, security, intuition, and peace.

Fear and Unease

Lay your hands on the Head Positions One and Four (see pp. 60–1 and 66–7 for all head positions). This relaxes you and helps you to let go of negative emotions. Front Positions One and Three (see p. 62) on the front of the body give you strength, enjoyment of life, and trust. Back Position Three (see pp. 63, 71) strengthens your nerves and relaxes the adrenal glands. Let your hands stay in each position for five minutes, or long enough for emotional equilibrium to be re-established.

Mood Swings and Depression

Try Head Positions Two and Four to even out moods and lift your spirits. In addition, lay your hands on the Front Positions One and Three and, for at least ten minutes, on the Back Position Three. The head positions balance the functions of the pituitary and pineal glands, which themselves govern hormonal balance. There is also an increase in the secretion of so-called endorphins, the body's own "happiness hormones". The Front Positions One and Three promote our feelings of self-esteem and we can connect more readily with our inner power.

Intensive Mental Work

If you face a mental challenge such as making a speech, try Head Positions Two and Four to activate the short- and long-term memory.

If you feel nervous, place one hand on the Solar Plexus (Third) Chakra and the other on the Third Eye (Sixth) Chakra (see Harmonizing Chakras, pp. 86–7). A surplus of energy in the head can then be integrated into the solar plexus. The energy harmonizes itself on a rational and emotional level, promoting relaxation and dissipating fear.

Stress and Worry

Whenever you are under stress, apply the Back Position Three over the kidneys. This is the seat of the adrenal glands, which produce the stress hormone adrenalin. When you treat yourself in this position with Reiki, you relax and relieve the pressure on the glands, slowing the production of adrenalin. If you often tend to worry, you should give yourself a treatment every day. This will strengthen your confidence and self-esteem. You may also try Head Positions One and Two, Front Position One at the center of the chest, and Back Position Three over the kidneys. In this case, remain for five to fifteen minutes in each position.

If you use Reiki regularly, ideally everyday, you will find it far easier to develop a clear, positive attitude to yourself and to life in general.

Insomnia

If you can't get to sleep at night or are generally wakeful, give yourself a treatment every day. Head Positions One, Two, and Four help you to switch off and to go to sleep more easily. You may also lie on your side in the so-called fetal posture (see also Sleep Help position, p. 51).

"Reiki is such a gift. It has helped me so much. I am calmer, my intuition is sharper and the world is now beautiful in my eyes."
DIANE

"My meditation has been most powerful and enriched by Reiki."
VALERIE

PERSONAL
RELATIONSHIPS

Reiki is a perfect means for becoming closer to others in your life. You not only can heal mental and emotional hurts and dysfunctions but also, over time, develop a special closeness with another person that was not there before.

The flow of Reiki energy can connect you more closely with your capacity for love and intensify your relationship with other people in general. Front Position One (see p. 68) activates the Heart (Fourth) Chakra (see p. 31) and enhances positive feelings of joy, happiness, and contentment. You begin to see your surroundings with eyes of unconditional love.

If you want to intensify and improve your relationship with someone, try the Heart Connection Exercise (see facing page). You can also use this exercise for preventing disputes and arguments.

Anger

When you are angry or in the grip of an uncontrollable temper (literally "seeing red"), lay your hands on the heart center (Fourth) Chakra, the Front Position One (see p. 62). Next, let your hands rest on Front Positions Two and Three (see p. 62). The contact with the Heart (Fourth) and Solar Plexus center (Third) Chakras (see p. 31) relaxes you, and allows your emotional and mental energies to come back into balance.

You may also lay your hands on the kidney region, Back Position Three (see p. 63). This calms and strengthens your nerves, allowing you to let go more easily. The techniques of the Second Degree (see pp. 52–3) are particularly supportive in the treatment of many kinds of psychological and spiritual problems.

By using the powerful, confidential Second Degree Symbols (see pp. 38–40 for the theory), you can use the healing energy that is generated in order to recognize the causes of underlying symptoms as well as for the elimination of deep-rooted mental and spiritual problems both in yourself and in others.

HEART CONNECTION EXERCISE

If you do this exercise together for a few minutes every day, both you and your partner will develop a stronger capacity for unconditional love. If you argue with your partner, try this exercise afterwards, if possible. You can also try it with children and, if you want to, you can carry it out in a reclining position, facing each other. Some people like to have gentle music playing in the background.

1. Sit face to face so that you can both easily reach your partner's Heart (Fourth) Chakra, at the center of the chest.

2. Lay your right hand on the Heart center of your partner. Lay your left hand over his or her hand.

3. Now gaze for a while into each others' eyes. After two or three minutes, both of you should close your eyes. You may feel a strong sense of love and unity. Stay as long as you like in this position — perhaps for 15 to 20 minutes.

"I felt a glow of light and love and joy beginning to open up within my heart center. The energy radiated all through me, entering all parts of my being, touching me, opening me, healing me."

PAMELA

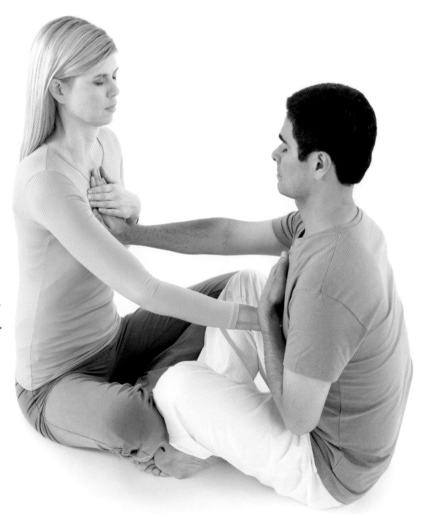

USES FOR
REIKI

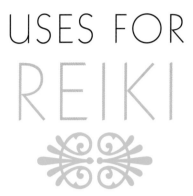

With the help of the techniques of the Second Degree (see pp. 52–3), you can amplify the flow of Reiki energy many times. With the help of the techniques of the Second Degree, you can amplify the flow of Reiki energy many times.

Room Cleaning

You can use Reiki energetically to charge and cleanse objects and rooms. This is very useful when you are travelling and have to stay overnight in hotel rooms, or whenever a room you are in seems to be filled with negative energy. With the help of the Universal Life Energy, amplified by using the First Symbol (see pp. 38–40 for theory), you can cleanse the room's atmosphere of negative influences and fill it with harmonious vibrations. This is a good way to cleanse your session-room before starting treatment.

Objects

As matter (objects) really consists of condensed vibration, you can give Reiki treatment to even the most everyday things, such as malfunctioning cars, jammed locks, machines, and gadgets. Reiki often helps when things don't appear to be broken but simply refuse to work.

Enriching Food and Drink

You can also enrich your food and drink with Reiki power and increase its nutritional value. If, for example, you often eat in restaurants, you can change the vibration of the food and cleanse it by using the First Symbol and, at the same time, holding your hands over the food for a short while. Using the same Symbol, you can also use Reiki when preparing food, for example when baking bread or tossing a salad.

Enhancing Energy

You can increase the available energy during a Reiki treatment by using the First Symbol before placing your hands on the body. Use the Symbol on areas where you want to enhance the energy flow or even before each hand position.

Personal Protection

In everyday life you can also use the First Symbol as protection against outside energies.

If you feel energetically oppressed or disturbed by other people, for example in crowded rooms, at public events, or in buses and trains, you can visualize the Symbol in front of you and energetically construct a protective screen.

Centering

Before each treatment center yourself with the help of the First Symbol, drawing it in front of you. This not only centers you but also makes you aware that you are a channel of Universal Life Energy.

Meditation

Using Reiki, you can enter a wonderful state of meditation. Reiki simply touches deeper layers within and puts you in touch with that part which is also described as the core of your being, or soul. Here you contact your source and feel connected with the whole. You can also use the powerful First Symbol to bring more awareness to your meditation. This creates a higher vibration of light energy around you, making it easier for you to raise the level of your consciousness and to observe your body, thoughts, and feelings. In meditation, you let go and relax. You allow yourself to fall into your innermost being; a state of absence of wanting and an absence of doing. In meditation, you experience moments of silence and peace. The Peace Meditation (see p. 113) puts you in touch with your Heart (Fourth) Chakra, or center.

Treating crystals and minerals

You can treat minerals, such as crystals, precious stones, and jewelry very effectively with Reiki. When you wear the jewelry it becomes an added source of positive energy. Hold the object under cold running water for a couple of minutes or so and then lay your hands over it. If you use the First Symbol for energy amplification, the minerals very quickly recharge themselves with positive energies.

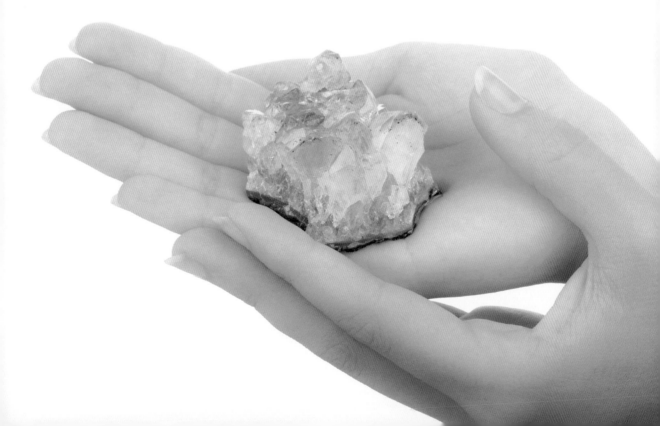

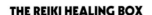

THE REIKI HEALING BOX

Using the appropriate Reiki Symbols (see pp. 38–40 for the theory), you can give healing simultaneously to several themes, people, and problem areas by using the Reiki Healing Box. This is a small box made of wood, cardboard, or any material other than metal. You use all three Symbols in order to send amplified healing energy (on all planes) to a person, an unresolved theme (perhaps an event from childhood), or a difficult situation.

1. Write the theme of your healing or the name of the person on a piece of paper and charge it with healing energy using the Symbols. You can use a photo of a person if you do not know him or her personally.

2. Treat each theme and each person individually and then put the piece of paper or the photographs, in the box. Allow Reiki energy to flow into the box.

4. Give Reiki to the healing box every day for a week. After a week, reconsider the urgency of the themes once more and, if necessary, recharge the box energetically with Symbols.

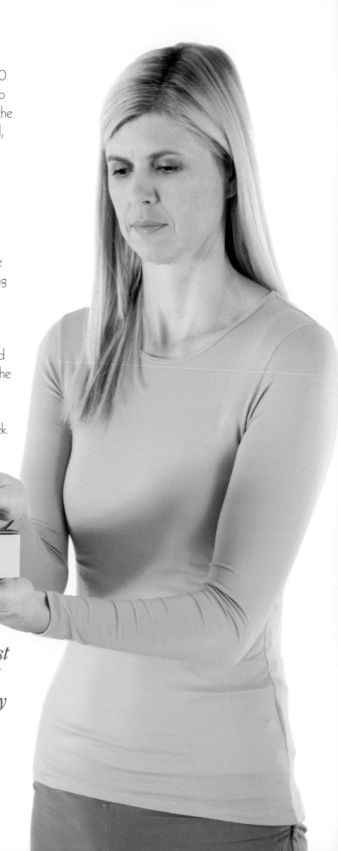

"With Reiki I found the innermost core of my being, something I had not experienced before. I suddenly knew me, and also that nobody could take that away again."
MARIANNE

Reiki and Other Therapies

The Reiki technique can be very successfully combined with other therapies. It activates natural healing energy in us and in others and is completely safe. Many therapists supplement and intensify their work with Reiki energy. Reiki can be combined excellently with massage, shiatsu, acupuncture, acupressure, chiropractic, Aura Soma color therapy, Bach Flower Therapy, homeopathy, breath therapy, polarity, Rolfing, cranio-sacral therapy, hypnosis, foot reflexology, aromatherapy, cosmetic massages, and many more complementary healing arts.

As we always touch with the hands in body work such as massage, acupuncture, or chiropractic, Reiki automatically flows into the receiver with each treatment. This kind of touching is often felt much more intensively by the receiver, whose personal experience also extends to the emotional and mental spheres.

Therapists

Some Reiki practitioners who also work as massage therapists and aromatherapists report that their work in those fields has positively changed and intensified since taking the Reiki First Degree. Many therapists feel that their therapy has become more holistic and involves more than just the physical plane when they supplement their practice with Reiki. They find that giving treatments is more enjoyable and the givers themselves are in much better contact with their intuitive side. The givers sense exactly what is best for the receivers in the moment and no longer exhaust themselves so quickly. They can also let their hands rest for longer on parts of the body. A massage therapist is also better protected by Reiki from the absorption of possible negative vibrations from the patient.

Many other therapies can also be used together with Reiki. If you work with people, no matter whether as an aromatherapist, rebirther, or psychologist, the use of Reiki energy always creates a harmonic framework in which the individual healing and growth processes often proceed with less effort and more effectiveness. Be ready to experiment and apply the Reiki energy in your own specialist field. Perhaps you will discover your own personal form of healing.

Massage

Reiki is ideal for combining with massage. Reiki itself is not a massage technique and you should not apply pressure or use circular motions in its practice. Here are a few suggestions for combining Reiki and massage. They are intended for professionals, using recognized massage techniques. If you are trained in massage, try these out, if not please refrain from their use.

At the start of the massage treatment, you can generally begin with Head Position One (see pp. 66–7 for head positions). This relaxes the receiver and directs energy inward. Then massage the sides of the throat and the nape of the neck for a few minutes. Also massage in the region of the medulla oblongata and, with circling motions, along the bone at the back of the head.

Next, you can use Head Position Four and hold the head. You may notice how, after a few minutes, the receiver relaxes more deeply and

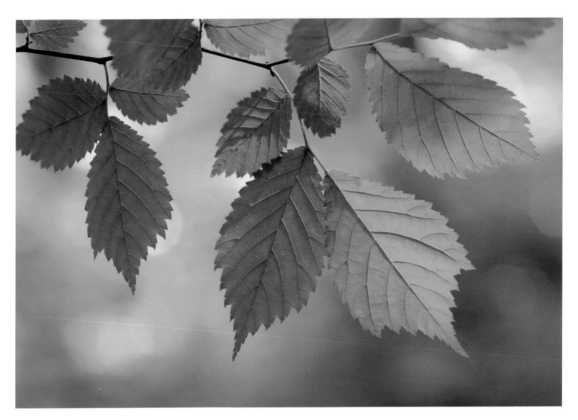

lets go of any tension. This position conveys trust and security. Now do a complete head and face massage the way you usually do it.

Then lay your hands on Head Positions Two and Three and let the Universal Life Energy flow in here. Now massage the whole front of the body, working from head to foot. Use a body oil to make your hands run more smoothly over the receiver's body. Whenever you feel like it, let your hands linger longer between the individual massage strokes and circular motions. You can also let your hands rest longer on parts you have already massaged. Trust your intuition and be led entirely by your hands. In this way, you will

"Reiki makes me slow down and rejuvenate. I love giving Reiki to my friends and family. It works!"
ALEXANDER

do exactly the right thing at the right moment. The physical blocks and energies released by the massage begin to melt and dissolve readily. Work your way down to the feet. Then ask the receiver to lie on his or her front. Now work upward along the backs of the feet and legs. After you have massaged the whole of the back, you can treat the back of the body with Reiki. Use Back Positions One to Five (see pp. 70–1).

At the very end, treat the knees and lay your hands on the soles of the feet. Treatment of the knees is important, because here we hold on to emotions and fears, including the fear of death.

We all fear the new and unknown and tend to be afraid of change. It is common to hold on to preconceived opinions, habits, and moods. Today, we go through so many radical changes (consciously or unconsciously) and our knees require a lot of support and energy. The feet are a very suitable point to end a treatment, because over the sole of the foot is a series of foot reflex zones which are connected to various organs and parts of the body.

A Reiki student reported that, after the First Degree seminar, she received an exchange treatment from a friend who practiced Reiki. When her friend touched her knees, there appeared to her all the forgotten pictures and memories of the death of her boyfriend, who had died unexpectedly a few months earlier.

The Reiki student had repressed this experience and now also remembered that she had been aware of increasing problems in her knees since her bereavement. Thanks to the Reiki treatment much of the tension in her knees was released. The pain completely disappeared and she found she was able to go for long walks again.

Allopathic Medicine

You can use Reiki very effectively with allopathic medicine as it enriches every form of medical treatment, always supporting the body's healing processes. Reiki does not reduce the effect of medication or other medical treatments, but supports the body through its detoxifying and harmonizing action. Reiki is not a substitute for medical treatments or drugs, but it can enhance their effectiveness. Reiki can be particularly useful in speeding the healing process when the receiver is very weak and sick, for example after a serious accident or an operation, and has to be treated with allopathic drugs.

As previously mentioned, Reiki can be used for First Aid (see pp.96–7) and before or after – but not during – an operation (see p.54). Reiki also supports the detoxification function of the kidneys and liver and helps the body to excrete toxic substances.

Psychiatric Therapy

Reiki can be used successfully in psychiatry. However, it is very important and advisable, especially in the case of patients with neuroses, psychoses, and personality disorders, to work in close consultation with the doctor responsible. He or she can point out possible complications which might arise in the treatment.

A man who was depressive and about to receive electrotherapy had heart problems and so was unable to take medication. While he was waiting for the results of a medical examination he became very tense and nervous.

A Reiki student offered him a Reiki session for relaxation, later reporting that she had never given Reiki to such a tense person. In the course of the treatment she was very pleasantly surprised to see how much he could let go and relax. Within a short period, he received two more Reiki treatments which greatly eased his fears.

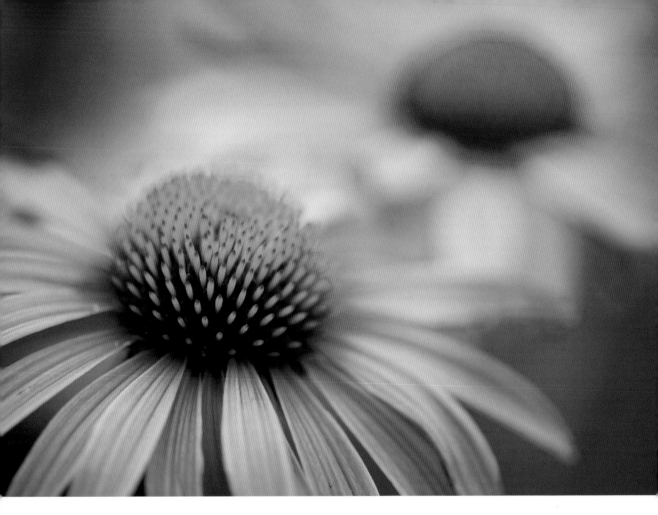

Hypnosis

The technique of hypnosis and the Reiki method complement each other well. A Reiki treatment can be given before, during, or after the hypnosis session. In so doing, you can simplify the direct contact of the receiver and the awareness of events in the past, present, and future. On the other hand a Reiki full body treatment can also be greatly intensified by hypnosis, as you can relax very quickly and profoundly in the hypnotized state.

If you have learned the technique of self-hypnosis, you will enjoy a completely new experience with Reiki. You can make a recording of your own voice for a hypnosis lead-in and then treat yourself directly. You can also use the combined effects of hypnosis and Reiki to concentrate on certain specific topics.

Hypnosis in combination with Reiki is particularly suitable for addressing themes such as depression, withdrawal symptoms from addictions, childhood traumas, eating disorders such as bulimia and anorexia, and various psychosomatic complaints. In addition you can also work generally with hypnosis on themes for many kinds of personal growth.

"Reiki has made me feel happier with myself. It has also allowed me to explore feelings I don't think I would have touched because I would not have known how to handle them. I feel safe now that I have a tool to use."

EMMA

Fasting

This is a traditional method which has recently become popular, that is used to cure a large number of illnesses, such as kidney and liver disorders, arthritis, asthma, digestive disorders, skin rashes, and high blood pressure. Reiki energy supports all types of fasting. It mitigates its unpleasant side effects and speeds up the elimination of the toxins which are released by the fasting. The Reiki energy also fortifies the immune system during this time of reduced nutritional intake. Ideally, you should give a full body treatment every day during the fasting period.

Bach Flower Therapy

This therapy was developed in the 1930s by the English physician, Dr Edward Bach. Using his intuition and sensitivity, he explored and discovered the healing effects of certain plants. He also established that the flower essences can harmonize conflicts on the mental-spiritual plane.

By a simple and natural method, he was able to capture the energy frequencies of flowers and conserve them in a flower essence.

He then observed that illnesses caused by an emotional imbalance or a false mental attitude disappeared shortly after the person suffering from such a malady took these flower essences.

Bach speaks of a mental-spiritual conflict which occurs when the person has lost contact with his soul, no longer receiving the fine impulses which can find expression, for example, through his intuition or conscience. When what a person's soul wants to express no longer accords with what his personality expresses, the person suffers from a mental-spiritual conflict and becomes ill. Each of the flowers discovered by Edward Bach vibrates at a specific energy frequency, corresponding to a positive energy frequency of the soul.

When we are in a blocked state, the personality can only receive the impulses from our soul in a distorted form, if at all. Then we suffer negative moods such as anger, depression, or fear. If, in such a state, we take the right flower essence, we can redirect our feelings positively.

Since, according to Bach Flower Therapy, a person's mental-spiritual blockages may have individually different effects on the physical plane, no specific flower essence can be assigned to a specific illness. It is much more important to find out, regardless of this illness, the nature of the mental-spiritual blockage of the person seeking advice and how this blockage expresses itself. It is in accordance with this that the Bach Flower therapist combines the correct flower mixture for the client. The essence is then taken in the form of drops for a period of about three to six weeks or longer.

With the help of Reiki, the treatment flask, specially composed for the patient, can now be enriched with Universal Life Energy. Because Reiki energy, just like flower essence, consists of subtle vibrations, these two methods support each other perfectly. Bach Flowers have a harmonizing effect on the mind, so they relieve the physical body. The combination of Reiki and flower therapy is very well suited, particularly for patients who are emotionally unstable and out of balance. The flower essences help to relieve fearfulness, inhibitions, traumas, and shocks by bringing them gently into the person's awareness so he or she can resolve them.

Bach Flower Therapy is used by many people for the prevention and self-healing of disharmonious mental and spiritual conditions. With Mental Healing, we can additionally harmonize and heal the emotions. In this process we can become aware of the underlying cause of the problem. The flower essences help us to balance our energies more easily.

Hold the Bach Flower remedy treatment flask in one hand and lay the other hand over it with the fingers closed. Let Reiki energy flow into the flask for a few minutes. You can use the First Symbol to make the Bach Flower mixture even more effective.

I treated a one-year-old baby with Reiki and Rescue Remedy drops (a mixture of seven different flower essences). As a result of a crisis in the parents' relationship and an attack of meningitis from which he had not yet completely recovered, the baby was physically and emotionally very weak and completely out of balance. According to the parents, the child was also a bit slow for his age. I trickled a few emergency drops into the child's mouth at the start of his treatment. He immediately relaxed and stopped crying. Then I treated both mother and child with Reiki. During the treatment, the baby seemed to recover from a profound exhaustion. I left the emergency drops with the mother to be taken daily for about the next four weeks. After a week, the mother phoned me to tell me that the child was much better. The fever and the blotches on his body, symptoms of the meningitis, had completely disappeared three days after the treatment. The baby also became bright and lively again and very quickly caught up in his development.

Aura Soma Colour Therapy

In the early eighties, Aura Soma Color Therapy was created by the English pharmacist, Vicky Wall. This form of holistic therapy combines the healing effects of colors, plants, precious stones, and perfumes. Vicky received the inspiration for the first Aura Soma essences while in a meditative state. Since she was blind, she was unable to see the brilliant colors which appeared as she mixed the ingredients together. The combined effect of the powerful colors, ethereal oils, and precious stone energies gives these substances an intense vibration.

We can well integrate the use of Aura Soma essences in a Reiki treatment. First we use a few drops of the essence on ourselves, waving it in our own aura. At the beginning of the treatment we smooth the reciever's aura from head to foot, spreading the essence into the receiver's aura. This has a cleansing effect.

PEACE MEDITATION

You can do this meditation either sitting or lying down — for example in bed as soon as you wake up or before you go to sleep.

1. Sit up straight and relaxed, close your eyes and let your breath flow naturally in and out.

2. Now put your right hand under your left armpit and your left hand under your right armpit. Relax and direct your whole attention to the chest area in between.

3. Allow a feeling of peace to rise from your heart. Just relax and direct your attention to this feeling.

4. When you are centered here and relaxed, you automatically come into contact with your inner peace. The heart becomes calm and sends out harmonic vibrations which you experience as love and peace.

5. Remain for about 10–15 minutes in this position, enjoying this feeling.

"I use Reiki to balance my own energies and nourish myself. Both the first and second degrees helped me on my spiritual journey."

MARK

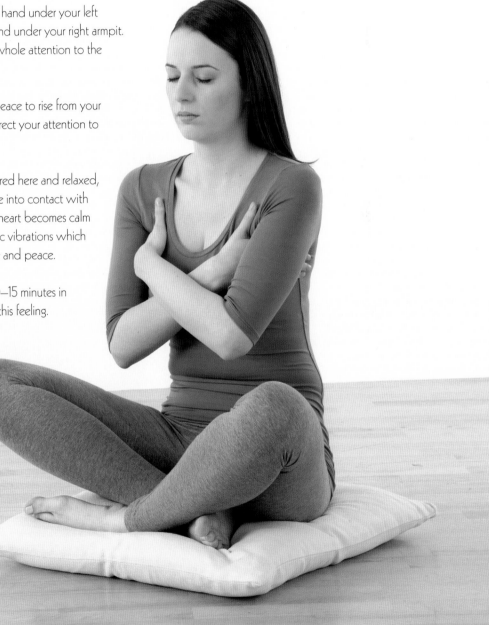

The Aura Soma essences which Vicky produced under spiritual guidance can be divided into three different categories: Balance Oils, which are applied directly to the corresponding part of the body; and Pomander and Master Quintessences, which are wafted into the aura. The term "aura" describes the electromagnetic field which surrounds each of us and which can be seen by people sensitive to it. By using a Pomander or a Quintessence, we can instill a specific color and therefore the healing vibrations of the Aura Soma essence into our energy field. The essences work through the subtle aura to produce their effect on the physical body. Colors trigger emotions. Blue has a calming effect and a powerful red always has a stimulating effect, while pink has a calming and nourishing effect on the heart.

By using a Pomander or a Quintessence, we can cleanse and heal the aura. When we apply the Master Quintessences, we additionally take the master energies into the aura and tune ourselves to these qualities. The "Lady Nada" essence, for example, helps us to transform negative energies into positive ones and reduces aggressions.

Reiki and Aura Soma make a good combination. You can use an appropriate Pomander or even a Quintessence at the start of every Reiki treatment for stroking the receiver's aura. You choose an essence intuitively or according to what you feel is appropriate for the receiver. For example, some people need the color green to allow more inner space and centering. After the treatment, you can cleanse yourself energetically using a Quintessence or a Pomander. The Quintessence "Serapis Bey" and the White Pomander are highly suitable for therapists for energetic cleansing between treatments. It is also helpful in Reiki seminars, especially before the energy transmission, to cleanse the aura with Aura Soma essences. It is a wonderful ritual for tuning in and for using before meditation.

Reiki for Health Professionals

The Reiki method is particularly useful to doctors, pediatricians, nurses, psychologists, non-medical therapists, physiotherapists, and all those who care for the elderly. Patients in intensive care units can also benefit greatly from Reiki. Babies and small children are very receptive to energies. Their senses have not yet developed the protective defence mechanisms of adults.

Years ago, I visited a friend in hospital. I walked down a long, sterile corridor in the ward and heard a baby screaming in the distance. As I saw nobody taking care of the baby, I approached the cot and held my hand a distance above the baby's head, level with the fontanelle. The baby immediately stopped screaming. I was astonished and pleasantly surprised at this rapid reaction.

Helping the Elderly and Sick

In the healing and caring professions, when normal human contact is important, physical touch, treatments, and massages gain a quite different quality when they include Reiki. Elderly and sick people benefit on many levels.

Older people in society often feel useless and shunted on to the "sidings". As our living conditions have changed so much and the typical family structure has gradually weakened, elderly people are often disoriented and do not feel valued, especially by the younger generation. Many live apart from their relatives in homes established just for that purpose. When their enjoyment of life diminishes, they become sick more frequently and, because of their condition, are then often bedridden. The Universal Life Energy of Reiki can nourish and energize such individuals.

For the elderly, Reiki can be given in a sitting position (see pp. 78–81). It is a good idea to make the treatment shorter than usual – about twenty to thirty minutes. Even though the body always takes up as much Universal Life Energy as it needs, a long Reiki treatment may put a strain on an elderly person. Sometimes, even holding the hand of a person needing help or laying your hands on the shoulders for a while is enough, as Reiki flows with every contact.

Reiki for the Dying

In today's society, dying and death are still subjects surrounded by strong taboos, though this is gradually changing. We are afraid to die and death is the worst thing that can happen to us. But death is part of life and is a natural process. It can be a totally fulfilling, liberating, and completing experience, regardless of when it comes for each of us. Birth and death are transformations into another form of existence. In death we leave the physical plane and our immortal essence, our soul, moves on to the next stage in its process of development.

With Reiki, you can give support and make this process of transition much easier for the dying person. You can hold the dying person's hand or treat him or her with Reiki energy. The person will feel protected and will find it easier to let go, or move into the other dimension. Reiki calms the person while allowing the natural process of dying to take place. It is also possible to accompany animals during death with the same kind of Reiki treatment.

"Two patients I treated became so relaxed, as though they were ready to finally let go. I sensed that they were very close to death and they were able to just slip away. They went into deep relaxation and stopped breathing."

A REIKI STUDENT WORKING IN A CANCER HOSPICE

REIKI
IN A GROUP

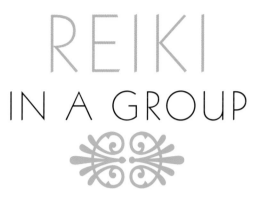

In group treatment, you can share the energy with other Reiki channels and friends. The treatment time is usually shorter than for a normal treatment. The Reiki power flows more intensely, the energy is made more active and the effect is appreciably stronger. In a group of five or six people, one person lies down and is treated by each of the others in turn.

Group treatments are especially effective if anyone has a severe illness, though for the best outcome one or more daily group treatments are usually required over a prolonged period, so a level of commitment from all the group members is required.

At the start of the treatment, the receiver's aura is smoothed by one person (see p. 65). One person can work on the head, while two others concentrate on both the left and right sides of the body. One of these should treat the inside of the thighs and the knees, and another the feet and soles of the feet.

Treat the front of the body for about ten minutes in this way, then ask the receiver to turn over and let healing energy flow into the back and the back of the legs for another ten minutes. At the end, one person should smooth the receiver's aura again. Take it in turns, so that each member of the group has a chance to become the receiver.

Small Groups

In a group with three people, one is the receiver, the second begins at the head, and the third treats the front positions. When the one being treated lies face down, the other two can treat the back positions, simultaneously treating the back from head to foot, also treating the knees and the soles of the feet. Both sides of the body are treated for about fifteen minutes. Then change over, so that everyone has a turn.

It is a good idea to play soft, meditative music and perhaps also burn oils in an aromatherapy burner to create a relaxing atmosphere.

The Reiki Sandwich

Another way to treat in a group of three is the Reiki Sandwich. Here, one participant sits in the middle and is treated simultaneously by both givers from the front and the back, or from the sides. Do the Reiki Sandwich in a sitting position and spend about fifteen minutes on the treatment. First, one giver smoothes the aura and then the hands are laid intuitively on certain areas of the body. To round off, smoothe the aura once more. Then change over so that each person receives Reiki in turn.

The Reiki Circle

This is ideal for using at short group meetings and during Reiki seminars – an effective way of activating and applying Reiki throughout a group. In this case, the giver is simultaneously a receiver. Stand or sit in a circle and lay your hands gently on the shoulders or the waist of the person in front of you. Allow the Reiki energy to flow through the hands.

Second Degree Work Group

You can also carry out group treatments using the techniques of the Second Degree (see pp. 52–3). In advanced Reiki courses, we join together to give group healing using Distant Healing (see pp. 54–5). The idea is to work directly on people, themes, or problem areas, with several people giving treatment simultaneously. We send healing to a specific situation and visualize positive qualities and energies to manifest for those involved.

Group support

Karin had requested support and healing before a job interview as she was feeling nervous. The group gave healing and visualized Karin's positive qualities. They visualized her handling the interview with a positive self-image and a self-assured manner. They marked the situation with a label showing the exact date and time of the interview. Karin related that she had never before been so calm and relaxed at interview, and was offered the job.

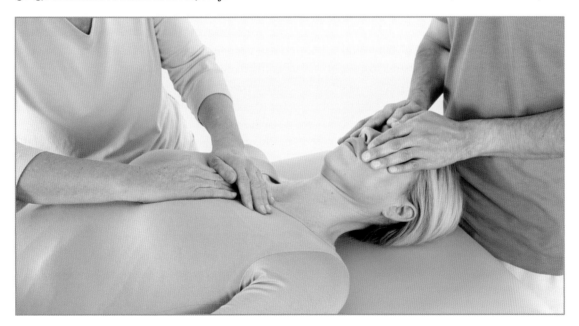

7. ON HEALING AND ILLNESS

When we are healthy, we feel strong, full of energy and the joy of life. We are balanced, contented, and in harmony with ourselves. If we "fall out" of this harmony our body creates an illness, or an imbalance. This kind of disturbance first takes place in the mind and is later mirrored as a physical symptom. The body is not sick; only the whole person can be sick, but this illness manifests as a bodily symptom. The body is a reflection of our mental state.

In order to understand the phenomenon of health and illness better, we must think of a person as a unit made up of body, mind, and soul. The body is the solid, earthly, material part. It is the "husk" of the soul, whereas the mind and the soul are "subtle". The mind connects us with an inexhaustible source of light, love, and wisdom. The soul is connected to us through our Higher Self and knows our purpose in life.

"I have found my desire for spiritual peace, my sense of fulfillment has got much stronger and my determination to cure myself is greater."

DAVID

Bach's "Meaning of Illness"
The English doctor and founder of Bach Flower Therapy, Dr Edward Bach, pointed out that the presence of an illness always implies conflict between what the person wants and the life plan of the person's soul. Illness is the result of this conflict created when the person refuses to do what the soul really wants. The disharmony, or the illness, exists between the higher, or spiritual, Self and the lower personality.

Bach said that sickness is sent to us to speed our personal growth and that it is "benevolent" in nature. He describes illness as a method of bringing us back to the path of understanding. According to him, if we then followed our inner guide, we could live without illness. This has to do with our inner growth processes, which need not necessarily progress through the actual experience of illness itself.

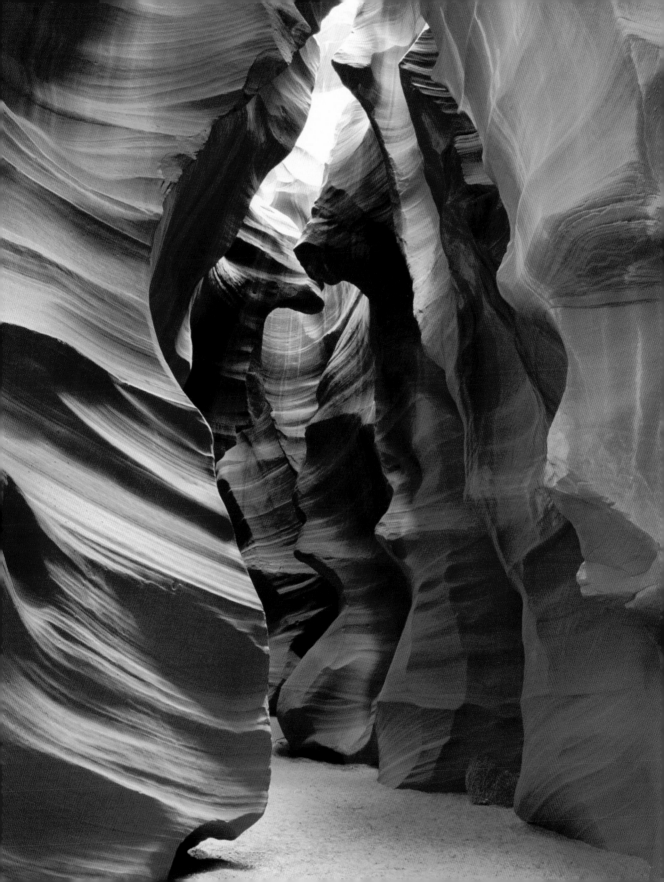

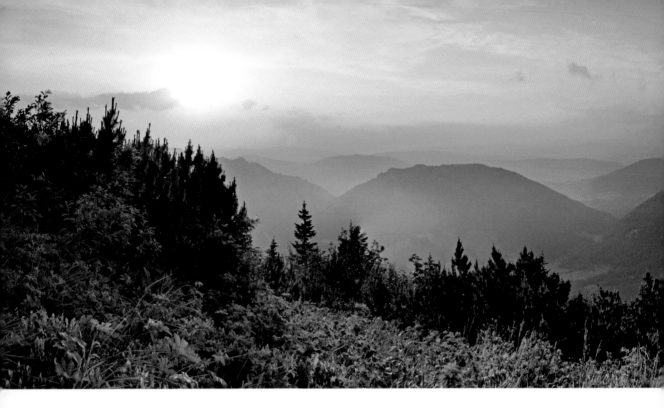

A person may feel physically healthy and free of the symptoms of illness, but still suffer from a disharmonious spiritual condition in the emotional sphere. If this person is unable to deal with the learning task on a mental-spiritual level, the process sinks to the physical level, evoking a reaction – which manifests itself as a symptom.

"I never imagined anything so powerful and wonderful could happen to me. I find Reiki helps me relax and has given me renewed hope that I may once again see perfectly."

SUSAN

Every illness is trying to tell us something and has a specific message for us. First, we must recognize and accept this message. When a symptom appears in a person's body, this is first experienced as a disturbance. The rhythm of our life and daily routine is interrupted. The symptom demands attention. It is most important not to reject and repress the illness, but to understand its signals. Through the physical symptoms something is shown to us. If we accept the challenge and are honest with ourselves, we can learn from it. We have taken the first step toward healing.

Transforming Belief Patterns

The cause of a sickness lies in the mental-spiritual sphere, and it is here that we must search for the first possible solutions in the recognition and transformation of our own

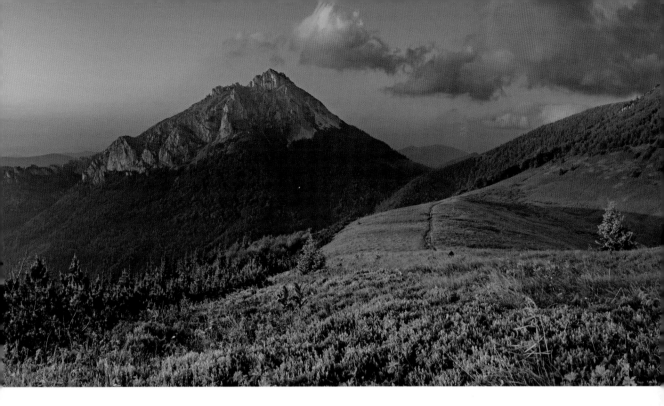

negative belief patterns and attitudes to life. Healing efforts directed specifically at the body are helpful and ease the pain, but they have no effect on the root of the problem. Through holistic, consciousness-expanding, and mental healing methods such as Reiki, spiritual healing, homeopathy, hypnosis, healing counseling, and healing meditations, we may be able to achieve a permanent cure. With Mental Healing (see pp. 82–3), we can work directly on the symptoms of sickness and their causes. We can clearly recognize what is wrong with the ill person, what has been repressed, and what he or she needs to become completely healthy again. In the healing process, suppressed feelings can also be activated. It is important that the person being treated accepts these feelings and allows them to express themselves.

We usually come very quickly to the actual central theme of an illness, by answering the following questions: "What does the symptom stop me doing?"; "What does the symptom force me to do?"; "What are the accompanying circumstances when it occurs?" For example, an attack of flu prevents you from accepting an invitation and forces you to stay in bed. In talking about your physical symptom, you might more easily understand what is behind it by paying attention to how you express yourself and the language you are using. This may point you in the right direction and you may be able to recognize the root cause of a symptom. For example, if an office worker dares not admit to herself or to her boss that she is fed up and would like to take a few days off, her physical body might act by catching a cold. On the physical plane, however, the

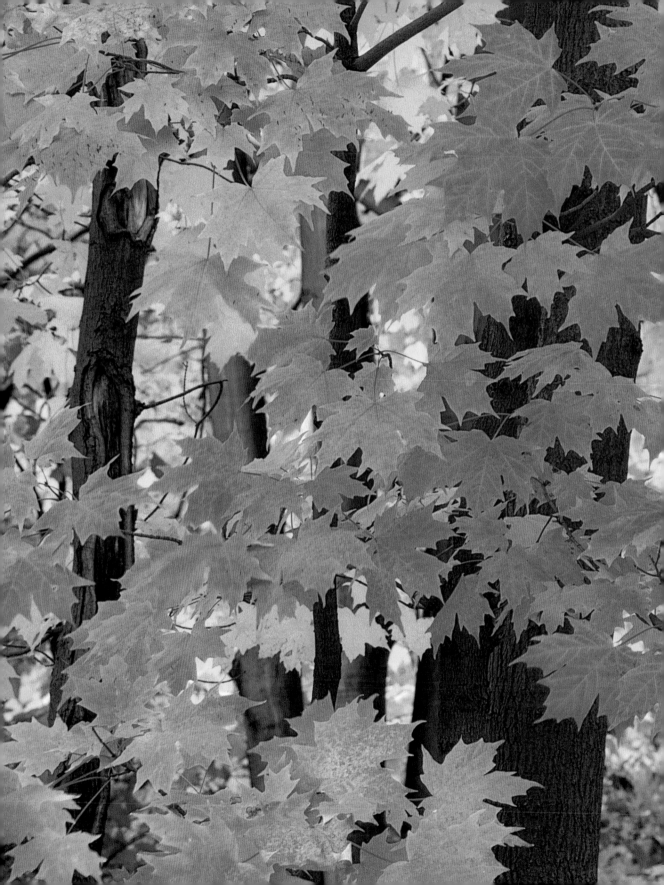

blocked nose is accepted and leads to the desired result. In this way, the unconscious wish manifests itself in the body and uses the cold as a symptom in order to make the actual wish conscious.

Sensing Messages

Before a problem in the body shows itself as an illness, it announces itself in the psyche as a theme, idea, wish, or fantasy. If we are in contact with our Higher Self and our unconscious, we can sense their messages. If we give such impulses room and, as Dr Bach said, follow "the guidance of our soul", any imbalance will not go so far as to manifest itself in the physical sphere. If, however, we live according to narrow ideas and standards and do not pay attention to the messages of the soul and our unconscious impulses, the body tries to find a more direct, visible language. So, after an initial slight functional disturbance, an acute physical symptom, such as an inflammation, may develop. This symptom may settle anywhere in the body. As laypeople, we recognize these symptoms by their last syllable "-itis", as in arthritis or cystitis, for example. Each inflammation in the body is a demand for the recognition of something and an attempt to reveal an unconscious conflict.

"Since the Second Degree my therapy work has increased. I now know how to give healing with confidence."

DEREK

"All that is needed is to find your center and meditation is the simplest way to find it. It will make you whole, healthy spiritually..."

OSHO

Chronic Disorders

If these hints are not recognized and understood, the acute inflammation turns into a chronic complaint, such as any of the symptoms with the ending "-osis" – arteriosclerosis or osteochondrosis, for example. Chronic disorders often initiate slow physical changes which then, at a later stage, become incurable, such as cancer, organ degeneration, or AIDS. This development may then finally lead to death. So illness is a challenge which demands our further growth. When we recognize the messages brought by our symptoms, we have a chance to use them for our further development and healing.

The Experience of Healing

By respecting and loving our bodies and accepting ourselves as we are, we experience healing. We have to redevelop a feeling for ourselves and for our bodies in order to come more closely into contact with ourselves. In our society today, particularly in Western culture, the mind is dominant. In other words, we live much too much in our heads and do not pay enough attention to our bodies and our feelings. If we cut off from this source of energy which our feelings provide, we often fail to enjoy life to the fullest. We feel low and depressed.

Depression is an expression of repressed, un-lived feelings. It is our feelings which make us alive and bring us into contact with our needs. Sensing what we need in order to feel content, fit, and healthy brings us closer to ourselves and strengthens our will to live. Joy and the will to live supply us with sufficient life energy, so that physical illnesses are almost impossible.

We all have a healer inside ourselves. Our "inner healer" or "inner doctor" knows the answers and the correct healing methods for our problem. In a loving manner, the "inner healer" corrects everything in his own time and we can help him to do so by allowing him the space and time to do what he needs to do. There are therapies using "healing talks" which permit loving, intense contact with an organ. You regain a feeling for yourself, receiving information about the cause of the illness and what you can do to become healthier. Another way of talking to your body could be in the form of guided hypnosis and meditation.

The Impotance of Relaxation

In the personal healing process, the relaxation of body, mind, and emotions plays an important role. As the body is near the Self, the conscious relaxation of the body is the first step. This makes it easier to achieve the second step, the calming of our thoughts, and in the third stage, to allow the growth of positive emotions of love and peace which provide deep relaxation and fulfillment. When we are in contact with our hearts, it is also easier for us to come into contact with our being or essence. Here we experience moments of peace and silence which allow us to feel ourselves as a part of the great whole.

A very effective way of becoming relaxed, happy, and healthy is meditation. Osho, an Indian mystic, developed special meditation techniques for Westerners. These methods are partly dynamic and active and aim at relaxation of the body through activity. Our lifestyle often exposes us to stress and we are frequently unable to express our feelings spontaneously. With his meditation techniques, Osho draws attention to the importance of living out negative energies such as anger or frustration. So, in some meditation methods, there are phases of catharsis which free us of bodily and emotional blocks. Only when we have let go of these tensions are we in a position to relax the mind and the heart and gradually to come nearer to our center.

Staying Healthy

In order for us to stay healthy in everyday life, it is important for us to remain in harmony with ourselves. A daily self-treatment with Reiki supports this process. With the Reiki Second Degree (see pp. 52–3), Mental Healing techniques (see pp. 82–3) are available to us and we can work even more effectively on personal themes, problems, and the causes of illness.

Through meditations and healing "conversations" with the body, we can further intensify inner growth and healing. Osho says the word 'meditation' and the word 'medicine' both come from the same root. Medicine means that which heals the physical, and meditation means that which heals the spiritual. Both are healing powers.

TALK TO YOUR HEART

You may find the following exercise valuable in helping you to reconnect with your feelings. Remain silent and become still. Concentrate your attention on your heart. If you sense a heaviness or constriction in the heart, try sighing to gain relief. This relieves pressure on the heart, releasing worries, fears, and anything you are hanging on to. Try this exercise to release worries and the day's tension before going to sleep.

1. Connect with the heart and place one or both hands on the middle of the chest (the heart center or Heart/Fourth Chakra).
2. Now start talking to your own heart as if it were an old friend.
3. Ask a question, if you like, and wait to receive an answer.

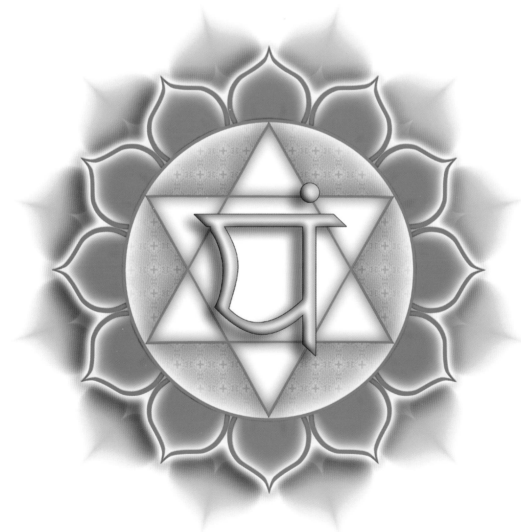

THE NADABRAHMA
MEDITATION

The following mediation, "Nadabrahma" (originally practiced by Tibetan monks and developed by Osho), has a powerful, calming, and healing effect. It can be carried out at any time of day, either alone or with others. If you practice it in the early morning, it is advisable to follow it with a pause of fifteen minutes before starting your day's activities. This meditation takes an hour and has three phases. The first two phases of the meditation are accompanied by relaxing meditative music.

Phase One (30 minutes)

1. Sit in a relaxed position with eyes and mouth closed.

2. Start to hum so that you can hear yourself easily and let the vibration spread through your whole body. Imagine your body is hollow inside like a pipe and is completely filled by the vibration of your humming. You do not need any special breathing technique for this meditation; just make a humming sound when you breathe out. You can also change the pitch or rock your hips gently if you feel like it.

Phase Two (15 minutes)

The second phase is split into two sections of seven and a half minutes each.

1. Hold both hands in front of your body (near the navel) with palms facing upwards.

2. Now move your hands in a circular movement away from your body. Your hands move forward away from your navel, then separate in two large symmetrical circles to the right and to the left. Carry out this entire movement in slow motion, so slowly that it sometimes seems as if your arms are not moving at all.
Feel inwardly how you are giving out energy to the universe.

3. After seven and a half minutes, turn your hands over so the palms are facing downward. Now move your hands in the opposite direction. Your hands meet near the navel and then separate again on both sides of your body, tracing large similar semicircles. Feel how you are receiving energy. If you want to, gently move your body, too.

Phase Three (15 minutes)

Sit or lie on your back and remain absolutely still and silent.

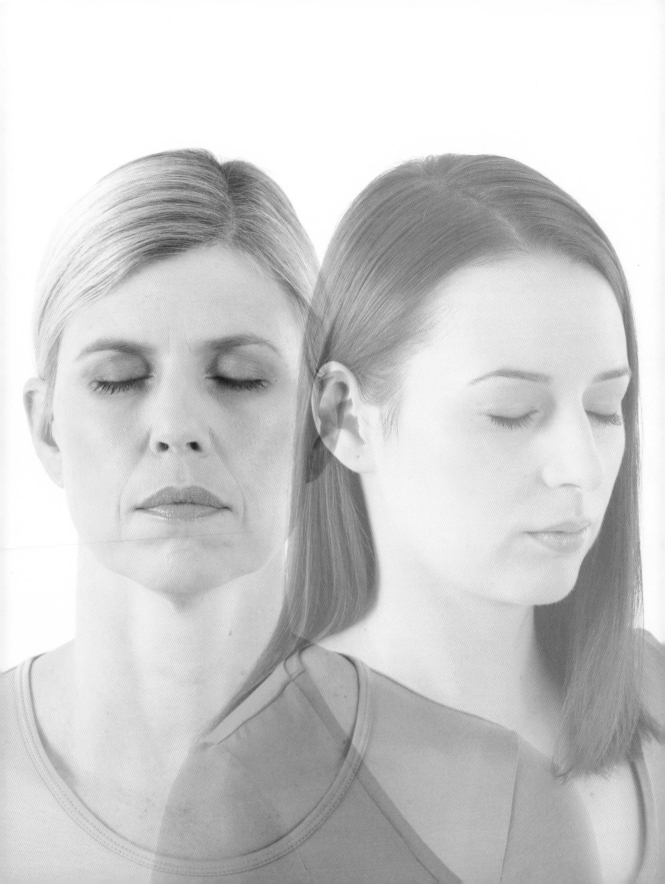

8. REIKI REPORTS

In this last chapter, I would like to share with you the widely varying experiences of some participants in my seminar courses. In these reports from Reiki channels and practitioners it is only too clear how much relaxation, healing, and positive change Reiki has brought into their lives. I sincerely hope that these impressions will bring Reiki nearer to you.

Treating the Elderly

"I treat many elderly people – aged 80 years and over – and they love it. The warmth stays with them and the pain lessens. I have one lady who has arthritis and osteoporosis, as well as high blood pressure and heart problems. I have given her four treatments so far. Her shoulder, neck, and the back of her head get very tender and even touching in light massage hurts. Reiki is wonderful. I can use it to give pain relief and increase mobility in her neck. She doesn't have to get undressed, which in itself can cause discomfort.

Another lady has been coming to me, as an aromatherapist, for about eight or nine weeks. She has lower back pain and pain in her leg. She's a keen walker but has been unable to walk for 18 months. Massage had helped. I've given her two Reiki treatments so far and she's walking again, her back is stronger, the pain is less, and she comes in smiling and happy. I've also found that by combining Reiki and aromatherapy, relaxation is very deep. Much deeper than I get with aromatherapy on its own. Muscles relax under my Reiki hands. It's wonderful, it's exciting, it's awe-inspiring. Sometimes I can hardly believe what's happening under my hands."

EILEEN

"It feels as if an even bigger change has been triggered, beginning to open me to receive love, attention, and care."

ALEX

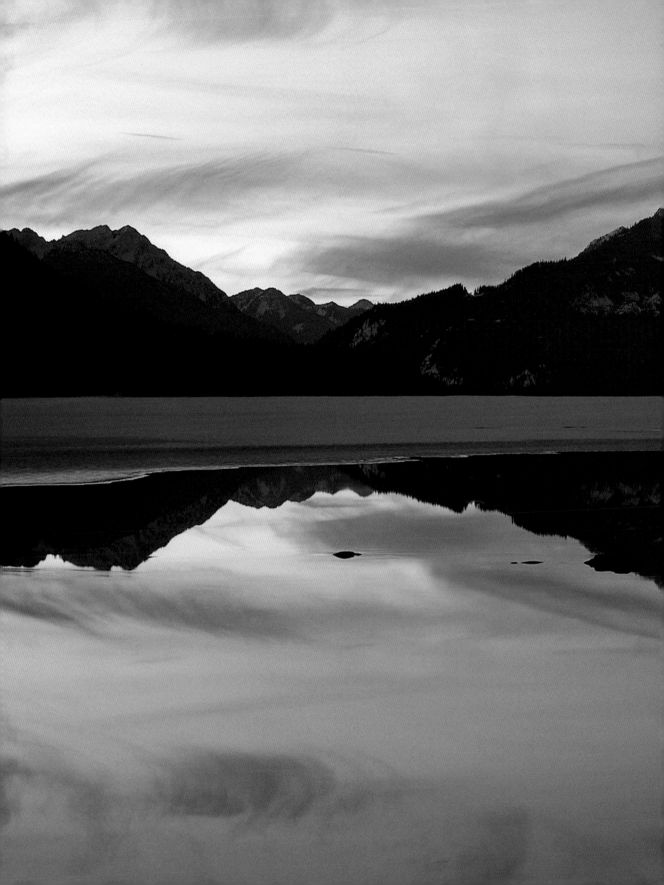

Treating Birds

"Birds respond wonderfully to Reiki. Whenever a bird flies into our house and has to be rescued, I first approach it using Distant Healing to calm it down. When it is quiet I go gently to it, cup it in both hands and carry it to the nearest exit. I then let it sit on my hand so that it can fly away. I frequently find that the bird has become so calm that it is quite happy to sit quietly for a short time before flying away. I have even known a small finch to sit and preen itself in the palm of my hand before taking off!"

AMANDA

Helping ME and Depression

"I have had ME/fibromyalgia for the past 11 years although, until two years ago, the more physical symptoms were masked by recurring severe depression. Until last year I had taken Lithium since 1990. I also take a battery of vitamins and eat a mainly vegetarian diet. For the previous four years I have been a non-smoker and since last year, following an adverse reaction, a non-drinker. Paula has used aromatherapy on me with mixed success. The oils seem helpful, but I find it hard to remain relaxed on the couch during a massage.

Sandra gave me my first hands-on Reiki treatment. I relaxed completely and stayed on the couch for over an hour. Indeed I had no sense of time at all and this is a feature of the treatment. I find that initially, I clear my mind of any problems, then relax completely. I have always felt very much better after treatment. Not only more relaxed but I seem to have much more energy. Possibly the greatest benefit, although there has been no improvement to symptoms, has been in attitude. I seem to have adopted a much more positive approach and, dare I say it, I seem to be more laid back.

From the treatment point of view there was definitely more heat from Sandra's hands after the Reiki attunement. One thing which has struck me is that when she covers my eyes her hands tend to feel cold, yet I can also feel the heat in my eyes – rather like lying in the sun with one's eyes closed. Both of us have noticed that I usually have little tremors or muscle jerks during treatment."

GEORGE

Experiencing Change

"I experienced a very deep sense of calm and peace that weekend [Reiki First Degree seminar weekend]. I felt that I had entered a very special place within me and felt certain that Reiki was a welcome addition to understanding my life.

My use of Reiki at the present is mainly in support of my own growth and development. From my direct experience of life and from the information I have gained through my interest in astrology, the present time is one of considerable change. This is both in my deep inner levels of beliefs about me, others and the world and about how I approach and connect with others. I find such change and transformation scary at times as I leave behind my old ways of surviving and, with the help of others, reinvent my strategies for surviving and growing today.

At other times Reiki has helped me to bring to my consciousness things and realizations that have helped me understand why I am behaving or feeling a certain way. Sometimes choosing a different path or redirecting a belief is the first part of a new view on reality. I experience Reiki as helping me to travel down my new road by providing energy and fresh insight and helping me to let go of old, less healthy ways of being.

On a physical level Reiki has been a great way of relieving pain and assisting healing. This can be anything from a strain to an infection to an injury. I have used Reiki together with homeopathy and shiatsu as well as with more conventional medicine and I feel it works well with all of these."

SAM

A Revelation

"I discovered Reiki by chance through a friend who was going on a Reiki weekend course to learn how to help her beloved dog who had been diagnosed as having cancer. When she told me about the course I knew instantly that it was just what I had been looking for and thinking about for several months.

The weekend was a revelation, it was like coming home, finding a missing part of me – a part which I knew was there but did not know how to get in touch with. It was like being reconnected to a source and being made to feel more complete. There was such a tremendous sense of relief to be reconnected in this way. It was very exciting but at the same time calming, balancing, and so right for me.

After the weekend I found myself giving Reiki treatments to many people. They just seemed to appear, and with some very exciting results. All were amazed by the heat coming from my hands, the colors and visions they experienced, the relaxation and revitalization they received, and the relief from pain. I was also delighted to find giving Reiki has exactly the same effect of relaxation and revitalization on me.

After the second weekend my commitment and reconnection were strengthened and another dimension opened with the Symbols and Mental and Distant Healing. I feel very privileged to have been given this gift and to be able to share the experience of Reiki with others, both in giving and receiving."

HELENE

A Life-Changing Experience

"So, for me, at least, Reiki was life changing. It initiated a very painful experience (I doubt if I would have been so vulnerable without attunements and I certainly wouldn't have had that energy release) but the outcome will eventually be worthwhile. I think I've grown a lot "softer" – more kindly. I seek not to judge so much and I do genuinely seek to serve now, and also to trust the universe or the soul or whatever it is that motivates us.

I've used a little Reiki on other people and it has always been beneficial. I've alleviated some pretty bad headaches, restored lost energy, and actually opened a bottle of perfume which was so firmly closed (for years) that it was thought the only way to open it would be to have it cut open ... and who would bother? But I gave it a little Reiki every day for two or three weeks ... just a minute or two and visualized it opening and sent it a lot of love and one day, it opened."

SUSAN

Success with Distant Healing

"George, a polarity therapist, asked me to do some healing on him. He was having an allergic reaction to something and had been told by an osteopath that, as he was training in polarity that it could be his ninth dorsal that was causing the problem. So we agreed a time for Distant Healing and I was really happy to do it as I knew that he would give me good feedback. He is very sensitive and used to working with energy.

Well, I sent him healing four times. He could actually feel it, which was wonderful. The first time almost cleared his allergic reaction, which was a runny nose. The second one sent him to sleep. The other two turned his mood around – he had been feeling a bit low beforehand. His allergic reaction disappeared and has stayed away.

After that I was really quite excited about Distant Healing as I had proof that it worked. The thing that interested me the most, though, was that my hands are so much more sensitive during Distant Healing. I was able to pick up some problems, which wasn't happening in my hands-on Reiki. Distant Healing seems to be more powerful. Also, sometimes I find I can't move my hands away from a spot. It is almost as if they are glued there and then suddenly they are free. It is really fascinating. I assume the body I am working on needs more healing there and so I let the hands do what they feel is necessary."

DAVID

Healing Horses

"I have given Reiki to many horses and I was asked by a friend, Linda, if I could attend to her pony. I went to see Oscar – the vet had given up on him as he was not responding to treatment. Oscar, a small Shetland pony, was suffering from very bad arthritis. I looked at him standing in the center of his stable, knee deep in a lovely bed of straw, a wedge of fresh hay for him to eat and yet, he was surrounded by a sad, grey aura. He obviously found it difficult to move and seemed not to be able to take a step forward. All four legs were locked and he just hung his head. His breathing was rapid and he felt too warm.

I started with Reiki on his head and gradually moved down his body. Very soon he softened and lay down in the straw, where he stretched out and went to sleep. I then spent a little time giving Reiki to the stable, where a lot of negative energy had built up.

I visited Oscar for three consecutive days and gave the same treatment. By the third day he seemed so much happier. I then let nature take its course and visited and treated about once a week for three or four weeks. When I last visited he was back out in the field and he cheekily ran away from me. He eventually humored me by standing for three minutes while I gave him a treatment. I knew he was back to normal when he quickly turned, bit my bottom, and trotted off up the hill."

BOB

Healing a Farm Dog

"Brin is a farm dog and had been run over. Both his back legs had been broken. The vet had given him a week to see some improvement and he did not seem very optimistic that he would be a working farm dog again. The treatment I gave Brin usually lasted for about an hour, concentrating on head, legs and bladder (he wasn't passing water), then finishing off with normal hand positions. During one treatment I concentrated a lot on his bladder – that evening he passed water.

Brin improved daily. You can now see him running the fields, rounding up sheep."

SHEILA

Tension Headache

"One of my aromatherapy clients was about to go on holiday and would be flying for the first time. She phoned to say she had been suffering with a headache for three days, so I offered to try some Reiki on her. I wondered whether she was getting tense about the flight.

I had a postcard from her some days later to say that the headache had disappeared after the Reiki session and that she was having a wonderful time, even indulging in a helicopter trip over the Grand Canyon."

ELISABETH

Reiki for Plants

"One of my regular aromatherapy clients was interested in my First Degree Reiki certificate and I was pleased to tell her all about Reiki healing. She decided to try it and I gave her a combined aromatherapy and Reiki session. During our conversation I had told my client about using Reiki on plants and she said that she had a very sick Christmas cactus at home which could do with some help. The next day I had a phone call from this lady, who said that she had frightened herself when she got home. She had decided to try Reiki on her plant and put her hands around it as she had seen me demonstrate earlier that day. To her amazement she had felt great heat in her hands and had almost dropped the plant! She decided to try again the following day, but there was no longer any heat. She concluded that it must have come indirectly from the Reiki session she had had earlier in the day."

SUSIE

Treating Animals

"I would like to give you a few examples of how well animals respond to Reiki healing. Firstly, an example of a cow in great distress. She had had a very difficult birth with her first calf. After the birth, as sometimes happens, she could not stand up. Her pelvis was very badly bruised, if not damaged, and she could not use her hind legs. In all other respects she seemed to be fine. As she lay in the field with the farmer feeding and watering her daily, I decided to try to help her.

Every day I would go to her, first using Distant Healing as I approached, thus calming her to my presence. I then placed my hands on either side of the base of her spine for a few moments and gently stroked her hind legs. She seemed to enjoy this and always kept very still, almost drifting off to sleep. I treated her for about twenty minutes each day. Every time I stopped she would look round with soft eyes as if asking for more!

Gradually, as the days went by she began trying to get up, but her hind legs were still too weak to support her. However, she did not seem to be in any pain. After a while the farmer, seeing that she was getting stronger, began to help her by lifting her up on a hoist to give added support, enabling her to stand for a short time each day. Every day she seemed to improve, also becoming more positive, as if her will to live had returned. Reiki was definitely helping her, because after each treatment she began to try to get up by herself. Progress was slow. Unfortunately too slow for the farmer. Had she been allowed time we were sure that she would fully recover. Sadly this was not to be: she was put to sleep. The next example concerns my elderly Jack Russell terrier. She had developed a very bad case of gastro-enteritis. Everything she was given to help seemed to do nothing. She was losing weight fast and became very restless and distraught. The night was the worst time as she needed to go out about every fifteen minutes. Somehow the situation had to be calmed down.

I decided to give her Reiki. Keeping her in her bed with my hands firmly on the lower half of her body, which was very hot, I began to calm her. Each time she tried to struggle up I kept her there, stroking with one hand and filling her with Reiki healing with the other. The heat seemed to penetrate deep into her body, warming her internal organs and intestines. Finally she went to sleep. This was repeated the next day and gradually the pain and diarrhoea subsided. She was given more Reiki to restore her depleted energy and by the third day was fully recovered. The vet said this could not be possible without medication as her condition was so serious."

ROSE

A Peaceful Death

"I keep a few free range hens and went to feed them one afternoon. I was very upset to find one of them in obvious distress. Her comb had turned purple and she was gasping for breath. She was an old hen and I realized that she was dying but decided to try Reiki anyway. My hens are used to being handled, but on this occasion she became more distressed so I gently put her back under a shrub and left her there while I tried some Distant Healing from the house. My husband checked her an hour later and to our amazement she was back to her normal color and running after the corn he threw alongside the other hens. She was fine when we closed them in for the night, but we found her dead on the floor of the henhouse next morning. On this occasion the Reiki appeared to relieve our hen of all of her distressing symptoms and allowed her to die peacefully in her sleep that night."

VALERIE

Healing Shoulder Pain

"I had arranged with my grown-up nephew to send him some healing on his lower back, where he has been having a problem.

I went through the sequence and when I put my hands on his shoulders I experienced this really odd feeing. It felt as though my hands were moving backward and forward, almost like a kneading action. When it had calmed down I moved my hands closer to the spine and the feeling came back.

After I'd finished the treatment I phoned Roy and asked him if he'd had a problem with his shoulders – he said he had. They'd been very sore and had a deep ache in them. I asked him how they were now and he was rather surprised to say that they were better. The pain had gone."

ELEANOR

GLOSSARY

AFFIRMATION

Usually a phrase or word describing a positive condition which we wish for ourselves.

ATTUNEMENTS

Special initiations in the Reiki energy, also known as energy transmissions. These open a channel for the healing energies in the chakras.

AURA

The energy field surrounding the body; a subtle, invisible essence. The human aura can be rendered visible by Kirlian photography.

CHAKRA

Circular energy center in the human subtle body. There are seven main chakras and they are located in the etheric body. In this book they are known as: Root (First), Sacral (Second), Solar Plexus (Third), Heart (Fourth), Throat (Fifth), Third Eye (Sixth), and Crown (Seventh). The word "chakra" comes from the Sanskrit, meaning "wheel". On the physical plane the chakras coincide approximately with the endocrine system.

CHANNEL

A person whose inner healing channel has opened to the subtle energies of Reiki, so that they can flow through him or her, to be used for self-healing or for the healing of others.

DISTANT HEALING

Allows you to send healing energies and loving thoughts on a mental level over a distance. Similar to radio and TV signals, healing energy is sent as though over a "golden bridge".

ENLIGHTENED

Describes someone who has experienced and lives his or her own divinity, and has witnessed inner "light". The presence of an enlightened one is a constant, permanent selfless state. Also known as a mystic, guru, or saint, such as St Francis of Assisi, for example.

ETHERIC BODY

The energetic counterpart of the physical body, in which the chakras are located.

FOREHEAD CHAKRA

Also known as the Third Eye, this is responsible for clairvoyance, telepathy, and spiritual awakening. It is stimulated by meditation.

HIGHER SELF

The part of us which is divine. We receive guidance from it, for example in Mental Healing.

LIFE FORCE ENERGY

The vital energy of life in all living things.

LIGHT ENERGY

Describes the fact that in nature the basic substance of all things is energy and energy in its essence can be described as "light". In Reiki this light energy is activated from within.

MANTRAS

Words and sounds which set subtle energies in vibration. These are used in meditations and in Reiki energy transmissions.

MEDITATION

A state of "not thinking" – "the awakening of the inner witness". Meditation happens in the present and is an immediate state of "not wanting, not doing". It is the ultimate state of relaxation.

MENTAL HEALING

Healing through the mind, by the emission of gathered mental energy. Can also take place in the form of Distant Healing.

MERIDIAN

The name for energy lines running through the entire body which transport life energy to the organs. By stimulating a meridian we balance and activate the function of each organ.

MYSTIC

See Enlightened.

"OM"

Holy sound or mantra used in religious ceremonies and meditations.

REFLEXOLOGY

A massage technique treating parts of the bodily organs by massaging the soles of the feet, where the reflex zones of the organs are located.

SACRUM

Bone plate above the cleft of the buttocks.

SANSKRIT

Ancient Indian language.

SUBCONSCIOUS

The parts within us which are unknown to us. Containing repressed energies, memories, themes, belief systems, and fears. The subconscious largely governs our behavior.

SUBTLE BODY

The part of the body which is invisible to "normal" sight and charged with a higher vibration.

SUBTLE ENERGY

As above.

SUPERCONSCIOUS

A level within us which is conscious and full of light; corresponds with the Higher Self, which knows and sees things clearly. Also known as intuition or spiritual guidance.

SUTRA

Word from Sanskrit, meaning "thread", theorem, or text-book. Sutras are also used in contemplation.

SYMBOLS

A Symbol comprises a pictorial drawing and a name, or mantra. The Reiki Symbols work on the body's healing channel, setting it to vibrate, so increasing the vibrational frequency of the whole body.

THYMUS GLAND

A gland of the endocrine system, which, when activated, positively stimulates the human immune system.

UNIVERSAL LIFE ENERGY

The energy of Reiki.

VIBRATIONAL FREQUENCY

The frequency of the vibration of our vital energy, increased by attunement to Reiki.

BIBLIOGRAPHY

Bach, Edward, *Heal Thyself*, (C.W. Daniel
Company Ltd, UK, 1994)

Baginski, Bodo and Sharamon, Shalila,
Reiki – Universal Life Energy, (LifeRhythm,
USA, 1988);
The Chakra Handbook, (Blue Dolphin, 1998)

Dethlefsen, Thorwald and Dahlke, Rüdiger,
The Healing Power of Illness, (Element, 1997)

Griscom, Chris, *The Ageless Body*,
(Simon & Schuster, USA, 1992)

Hay, Louise, *Heal Your Body*, (Hay House, 1988);
You Can Heal Your Life, (Hay House, 1987)

Horan, Paula, *Empowerment Through Reiki*,
(Lotus Light Publication, USA, 1992)

Müller, Brigitte, Günther, Horst H.,
A Complete Book of Reiki Healing,
(LifeRhythm, USA, 1995)

Osho, *The Orange Book*, (Rajneesh Foundation
International, USA, 1983);
Meditation, The First and Last Freedom,
(Boxtree, UK, 1995);
Vigyan Bhairav Tantra, (The Rebel Publishing
House GmbH, Germany);
Beloved of my Heart (Rajneesh Foundation,
Poona, India, 1978);
From Medication to Meditation, (C.W. Daniel
Company Ltd, UK)

Weber-Ray, Barbara, *The Reiki Factor*,
Expositions Press, USA, 1983

TITLES AVAILABLE IN GERMAN

Bind-Klinger, Anita, *Heilung durch Harmonie*,
(Aquamarin Verlag, Germany, 1992)

Simonsohn, Barbara, *Das authentische Reiki*,
(Scherz Verlag, Germany, 1996)

Zopf, Regine, *Reiki, Ein Weg sich selbst zu
vervollkommnem*, (Weltenhuter Verlag,
Germany, 1995)

GUIDED REIKI SELF-TREATMENT CDS BY TANMAYA

Heal yourself with Reiki – 18 Stages for Self-healing,
(Prabhu Music, 2008)

Inner Healing – 11 Stages for Self-healing, (Prabhu
Music, 2003)

MEDITATION CDS BY OSHO

Nadabrahma Meditation (music by G. Deuter)

The Forgotten Language (Talk to your Body)

ACKNOWLEDGMENTS

AUTHOR'S THANKS

I want to thank my friend Peter Campbell for his creative and practical support during the time I was working on the manuscript. Thanks to Jo Godfrey Wood, who edited the text, became interested in Reiki, took the First Degree and became a Reiki channel. I would like to thank all my Reiki students who shared their experiences with me and allowed me to use their reports on healing studies as examples for this book.

PUBLISHER'S ACKNOWLEDGMENTS

Gaia Books would like to thank the following for their help in the production of this book: models, Diana Goie, Deborah Lacy and Carlos Gomez; photographer's assistant Philip Banks.

PHOTOGRAPHIC CREDITS

Russell Sadur/Octopus Publishing Group, apart from the following:

Alamy/Andreas von Einsiedel 95; INSADCO Photography/Martin Plöb 105; Oleksiy Maksymenko 31. Fotolia/Dirk Czarnota 125; HuHu Lin 24; Morphart/fotolia.com 21; icholakov 36–37; Piotr Skubisz 26. Getty Images/ Franz-W. Franzelin 39. Photodisc 9, 23, 129. Thinkstock/Comstock 119; Digital Vision 33, 43, 59, 122; Dorling Kindersley RF 85; Hemera 16; iStockphoto 4, 11, 13, 18–19, 25, 34, 48–49, 93, 96–97, 101, 108–109, 110, 120–121, 134–135; Jupiterimages 6, 15; Siri Stafford 130–131.

USEFUL ADDRESSES

Reiki Outreach International
www.reikiassociation.net
www.reikioutreach.com
(USA)
www.reikiauskunft.de
(Germany)
www.reikitraining.com.au
(Australia)

The Reiki Association (UK)
reikiassociation.org.uk

The Reiki Alliance (USA)
www.reikialliance.com

The Reiki Alliance (Germany)
www.reiki-alliance-deutschland.de

INDEX

Commissioning Editor: Liz Dean
Art Director: Jonathan Christie
Designer: Penny Stock
Art Direction (photoshoot): Penny Stock
Photographer: Russell Sadur
Editor: Jo Wilson
Picture Researchers: Jennifer Veall, Giulia Hetherington
Production Controller: Sarah Kramer